This book is due for return on or before the last date shown below.

D1351234

EVALUATING TREATMENT ENVIRONMENTS

RUDOLF H. MOOS

EVALUATING TREATMENT ENVIRONMENTS

The Quality of Psychiatric and
Substance Abuse Programs

SECOND EDITION, REVISED & EXPANDED

TRANSACTION PUBLISHERS
New Brunswick (U.S.A.) and London (U.K.)

Library of Congress Catalog Number: 96–38940
ISBN: 1–56000–294–8
Printed in the United States of America

Library of Congress Cataloging-in-Publication Data

Moos, Rudolf H., 1934–
    Evaluating treatment environments : the quality of psychiatric and substance abuse programs / Rudolf H. Moos. — 2nd ed., rev. and epanded.
        p. cm.
    Includes bibliographical references and index.
    ISBN 1–56000–294–8 (alk. paper)
    1. Psychiatric hospitals—Evaluation.   2. Substance abuse—Treatment—Evaluation.   3. Mental health services—Evaluation.
I. Title.
    [DNLM: 1. Mental Health Services.   2. Substance Abuse Treatment Centers.   3. Mental Disorders—therapy.   4. Outcome and Process Assessment (Health Care)   WM 30 M694e   1996]
RC439.M75 1996
362.2'068'5—dc20
DNLM/DLC
for Library of Congress   96–38940
                                                                      CIP

To my mother and father,
who told me I could
and
to Jean Otto,
a soul at rest

Contents

Preface to the Original Edition   xv

Preface to the New Edition   xix

1. Understanding Treatment Programs and Outcomes   1

Part I—Hospital Programs

2. The Social Climate of Hospital Programs   23

3. Monitoring and Improving Hospital Programs   45

4. Assessing the Implementation of Hospital Programs   69

Part II—Community Programs

5. The Social Climate of Community Programs   91

6. Monitoring and Improving Community Programs   109

7. Assessing the Implementation of Community Programs   131

**Part III—Determinants and Outcomes
of Treatment Environments**

8. Determinants of Program Climate   157

9. In-Program Outcomes: Satisfaction, Self-Confidence,
   and Interpersonal Behavior   177

10. Adaptation in the Community   199

11. Special Issues: Client-Program Congruence and the
    Health Care Workplace   215

12. Implications for Treatment and Program Evaluation   233

Appendix A: Ward Atmosphere Scale Scoring Key   253

Appendix B: Community-Oriented Programs   261
    Environment Scale Scoring Key

References   271

Author Index   291

Subject Index   299

List of Tables

Table 2.1. WAS Subscale and Dimensions Descriptions   29

Table 5.1. COPES Subscale and Dimensions Descriptions   97

Table 8.1. Associations between Institutional Context and
            Treatment Climate   160

Table 8.2. Associations between Physical Features, Policies and
            Services, and Treatment Climate   164

Table 8.3. Associations between Residents' and Staff Members'
            Characteristics and Treatment Climate   169

Table 9.1. Correlations between WAS Subscales and Patients'
            Satisfaction and Morale   180

Table 9.2. Correlations between WAS Subscales and
            Patients' Initiatives   183

Table 9.3. Dropout Scale Items and Scoring Key   191

Table 9.4. Discharge Scale Items and Scoring Key   197

Table 10.1. Community Tenure Scale Items and Scoring Key   202

List of Figures

Figure 1.1.   A Model of the Relationships between Program
              and Personal Factors and Patients' Outcomes   3

Figure 2.1.   WAS Form R Means for Patients and Staff in
              160 Programs in the United States   30

Figure 2.2.   Patients' WAS Form R Means for Fifty-Five VA,
              Fifty-Five State, and Twenty-Eight University
              Hospital Programs   32

Figure 2.3.   WAS Form R Means for Staff in Programs in the
              United States and the United Kingdom   34

Figure 2.4.   WAS Form I Means for Patients and Staff in
              Sixty-Eight Programs in the United States   44

Figure 3.1.   WAS Form R Profiles for Patients and Staff on
              Simon Ward   46

Figure 3.2.   WAS Form R Profiles for Patients and Staff on
              Rulster Ward   47

Figure 3.3.   WAS Form R Profiles for Patients and Staff on
              Sampson Ward   49

Figure 3.4.   WAS Form R Profiles for Patients and Staff on
              Norman Ward   50

Figure 3.5.   Real-Ideal Discrepancies as Seen by Patients and
              Staff on Lathrop Unit   52

Figure 3.6.   Initial WAS Form R Profiles for Patients and Staff
              in Damien Unit   62

Figure 3.7. Follow-Up WAS Form R Profiles for Patients and
Staff in Damien Unit   63

Figure 4.1. WAS Form R Profiles for Patients and Staff in
Peer Confrontation Program   73

Figure 4.2. WAS Form R Profiles for Patients in Therapeutic
Community and Relationship-Oriented Programs   79

Figure 4.3. WAS Form R Profiles for Patients in Action-Oriented
and Insight-Oriented Programs   80

Figure 4.4. WAS Form R Profiles for Patients in Control-Oriented
and Undifferentiated Programs   80

Figure 4.5. WAS Form R Profiles for Patients in Social Systems
and Comparison Programs   85

Figure 5.1. COPES Form R Means for Members and Staff in
Programs in the United States   99

Figure 5.2. COPES Form R Means for Members and Staff in
i rograms in the United Kingdom   101

Figure 5.3. COPES Form I Means for Members and Staff in
Programs in the United States   107

Figure 5.4. COPES Form I Means for Members and Staff in
Programs in the United Kingdom   108

Figure 6.1. COPES Form R Profiles for Members and Staff in
Harbor Lights   110

Figure 6.2. COPES Form R Profiles for Members and Staff in
Shady Glen   112

Figure 6.3. COPES Form R Profiles for Members and Staff in
Pathways—First Assessment   118

Figure 6.4. Real-Ideal Discrepancies as Seen by Members and
Staff in Pathways   119

Figure 6.5. COPES Form R Profiles for Members and Staff in
Pathways—Third Assessment   121

Figure 6.6. COPES Form R Profiles for Members and Staff in
Safehaven—Initial Assessment   127

Figure 6.7. COPES Form R Profiles for Members and Staff in
Safehaven—Third Assessment   129

Figure 7.1. COPES Form R Profiles for the Salvation Army and
Public County-Funded Programs   133

Figure 7.2. COPES Form R Profiles for the Aversion Conditioning
Program   133

Figure 7.3. COPES Form R Profiles for the Milieu-Oriented
Program   135

Figure 7.4. COPES Form R Profiles for Residents and Staff in
Second Genesis Programs (from Bell, 1983)   137

Figure 7.5. COPES Form R Profiles for Clients in Programs with
Professional or Paraprofessional Staff   143

Figure 7.6. COPES Form R Profiles for Residents in Therapeutic
Community and Relationship-Oriented Programs   145

Figure 7.7. COPES Form R Profiles for Residents in Action-
Oriented and Insight-Oriented Programs   146

Figure 7.8. COPES Form R Profiles for Residents in Control-
Oriented and Undifferentiated Programs   148

Figure 8.1. Determinants of Social Climate in Psychiatric and
Substance Abuse Treatment Programs   158

Figure 10.1. WAS Form R Profiles for Staff on High and Low
Community Tenure Units   204

Preface to the Original Edition

This book presents a new approach to the comparison and evaluation of treatment environments. I call it a social ecological approach with some misgiving, because new terms may lead to confusion as well as to clarification. But I believe that the basic focus and organization of this work are unique. I offer a new way of measuring and changing treatment environments, and I describe how to link these environments' characteristics to patients' adaptation and psychosocial functioning.

In brief, social ecology is concerned with the environment and how people adapt to it. The field deals with both the physical and the social environment. I define social ecology as the multidisciplinary study of the relationship between the physical and social environment and individuals' cognition and behavior. Primarily concerned with the assessment and development of optimum human milieus, social ecology provides a distinctive "point of entry" into relevant clinical and applied problems. As I see it, it combines basic research approaches with a dedication to resolving common human problems. For me, the quality of life for patients and staff in psychiatric treatment settings is as significant as the objective empirical and statistical results.

The social and behavioral sciences are now as ever in a state of rapid development. Certain of these developments have influenced me most. In my clinical work I quickly found that I could not understand, much less predict, the behavior of my patients in settings other than my office. Even a decade ago the research literature and my colleagues had convinced me that this was a common problem. I was dissatisfied then with trait conceptualizations of personality, much as others are now. I felt that behavior was influenced by situational and environmental forces to a much greater extent than was commonly recognized, at least by psychologists.

About six years ago I became convinced of the importance of developing new methods by which to understand the environment. I felt that more knowledge about the environment would enhance an assessment of the impact of environments on human behavior. My overall aim is to identify environments that promote opportunities for personal growth, simultaneously enhancing both physical and psychological well-being.

Two thrusts of this work are most important to me. First, research is utilized in a practical, applied manner. Our work illustrates not only that relatively "hard-nosed" objective research can be made interesting and informative to patients and staff, but also that they can use it to improve their treatment climate. In this sense the aim of our work is to improve the quality of life for patients and staff in treatment programs and, by extension, for individuals participating in a range of other environments.

Second, the distinctive conceptual and theoretical overviews that grew out of the empirical work should help to stimulate further work in this area. Most important, there are common underlying patterns in a wide range of social environments, and the different methods researchers have used to study human environments can be categorized into six broad types. My hopes and my fears are one: that this work and these concepts will encourage and stimulate their own replacement.

The most distinctive features of this book include: (1) the use of similar techniques for assessing the treatment environments of hospital and community programs on common dimensions; (2) the explicit emphasis on both subjective (i.e., satisfaction, morale, helping behavior) and objective (i.e., dropout, discharge, and community tenure rates) effects of treatment programs; (3) the emphasis on the clinical utility of evaluation data about programs as an aid to teaching, to planning new and innovative approaches to treatment, to identifying trouble spots, and to successfully helping patients and staff change their own social environments; (4) the preparation of guidelines for the development of more useful and more complete program descriptions; (5) an emphasis on cross-cultural applications and comparisons of treatment programs, with particular relevance to treatment programs in the United States and the United Kingdom; and (6) an integration of relevant research approaches in other institutions into the literature on treatment environments.

My intellectual debts are too heavy and too numerous to detail. My bibliographic citations give a limited idea of those who have most strongly influenced my thinking. The initial research was supported by NIMH Grant MH16026 and MH8304, by NIAAA Grant AA00498, and by Department of Veterans Affairs medical research funds. The work profited from active collaborations with Marvin Gerst, Peter Houts, Edison Trickett, and Jack Sidman. These individuals provided a rich, stimulating source of new ideas and ever-present challenges. Gordon Adams facilitated the early phases of work; Marilyn Cohen, Diane House, Susan Lang, Eleanor Levine, Martha Merk, Chris Newhams, Phyllis Nobel, and Karl Schonborn each completed many essential tasks. Jim Stein, Bill Lake, and Bernice Moos coordinated the computer analyses.

During the last two years of the project, Marguerite Kaufman, Jean Otto, Charles Petty, Paul Sommers, Robert Shelton, and Penny Smail carried out the bulk of the detailed work. David Mechanic and Richard Price read and competently criticized a draft of the first edition of the book. Their comments helped me improve and clarify several chapters. Marion Langenberg typed the initial chapter drafts, Susan Glebus and Marcia Insel typed the second drafts, and Louise Doherty and Susanne Flynn typed and organized the final drafts.

David Hamburg, Chair of the Department of Psychiatry and Behavioral Sciences at Stanford University, deserves special recognition. For more than a decade he provided the supportive social milieu in which this work flourished. George Coehlo luckily recognized the potential of the work and was instrumental in helping me obtain initial funding.

Bernice Moos contributed to the compilation and statistical analysis of the data. Without Bernice, Karen, and Kevin, I might unhappily have finished this book somewhat sooner. They interrupted me, teased me, annoyed me, infuriated me, gumbled and gamboled—and thereby brought me joy.

Rudolf H. Moos
July 1973

Preface to the New Edition

When I wrote the preface to the first edition of this book I did not imagine that, after twenty-three years, I would be revising and updating the material. But, as luck and chance have it, many of the ideas I set out then are important and timely now. There is renewed focus on the overall quality of mental health care, on the process of care, and on the connections between the process and outcome of care.

The procedures we developed to assess the treatment environments of hospital and community programs have been widely applied in the United States and in other countries. As described here, they have been used to monitor and improve treatment programs, to assess the adequacy of program implementation, and to understand the determinants and outcomes of specific aspects of treatment environments.

The conceptualization of three underlying sets of treatment climate dimensions—that is, relationship, personal growth, and system maintenance dimensions—has been used widely to describe specific treatment programs and to contrast hospital with community programs and psychiatric with substance abuse programs. It also provides a framework to help integrate findings on the differential outcomes of treatment programs and on the results of client-program matching.

Over the past two decades, my research in this area was supported by NIMH grant MH28177, NIAAA grants AA02863 and AA06699, and Department of Veterans Affairs medical research funds. Most recently, the research and preparation of this manuscript were supported in part by the Department of Veterans Affairs Health Services Research and Development Service and Mental Health and Behavioral Sciences Service.

Elizabeth Burnett conducted bibliographic searches and expertly abstracted many publications, some of which were quite long and complex. She developed a practiced eye for finding and succinctly summarizing key points; she also provided valuable help with editorial tasks. Molly Kaplowitz conducted statistical analyses on new data that were drawn from Christine Timko's sample of psychiatric and substance abuse programs. The findings obtained from these data, which are described in chapters 7 and 8, enhance the current relevance of the work.

Bernice Moos contributed to the statistical analyses reported here; more important, she provided the social climate in which I flourished. Fortunately for me, after more than three decades, she is still coping effectively.

Rudolf H. Moos
July 1996

1

Understanding Treatment Programs and Outcomes

Three assumptions guide our approach to understanding psychiatric and substance abuse treatment programs and their outcomes. First, in order to examine the influence of treatment programs on patients' adaptation, we need systematic ways to measure the key aspects of the treatment process. Although most behavioral scientists endorse the idea that both personal and environmental factors determine behavior, evaluation researchers have typically conceptualized the treatment program as a "black box" intervening between patient or staff inputs and outcomes. Thus, these programs often are assessed only in terms of broad categories, such as the level of care provided or whether they accept patients with severe psychiatric disorders. To enrich understanding of these settings, we describe some useful ways to measure program characteristics; these measures enable us to identify specific aspects of treatment programs and to analyze their influence on patients' in-program and community adaptation.

Our second assumption is that although treatment programs for psychiatric and substance abuse patients are diverse, a common conceptual framework can be used to evaluate such programs, and doing so has several advantages. The framework allows us, for example, to identify similar processes occurring in different types of programs and to specify the extent of environmental change an individual experiences when moving from one type of setting to another, such as from a hospital to a community facility.

Our third assumption is that more emphasis should be placed on the process of matching personal and program factors and on the connections between person-environment congruence and patients' outcomes. To understand the influence of treatment programs more fully, we need to examine the selection processes that affect how patients are matched to programs. We also need to focus on how treatment environments vary in their impact on patients who differ in their level of impairment and the chronicity and severity of their disorders. Although researchers have recognized the complexity of person-environment transactions, empirical work has not adequately reflected the multicausal, interrelated nature of the processes involved.

Conceptual Model

The conceptual model shown in figure 1.1 follows these guidelines and provides a framework for examining treatment programs and how they and their patients mutually influence each other. In this model, the connection between the objective characteristics of the program (panel I), patients' personal characteristics (panel II), and patients' adaptation in the community (panel V), is mediated by the program social climate (panel III) and by patients' in-program outcomes (panel IV). The model specifies the domains of variables that should be included in a comprehensive evaluation.

The objective characteristics of the program (panel I) include the program's institutional context, physical design, policies and services, and the aggregate characteristics of the patients and staff. These four sets of objective environmental factors combine to influence the quality of the program culture or social climate (panel III). The social climate is part of the environmental system, but we place it in a separate panel to highlight its special status. The social climate is in part an outgrowth of objective environmental factors and also mediates their impact on patients' functioning. In addition, social climate can be assessed at both the program and the individual level.

Personal factors (panel II) encompass an individual's sociodemographic characteristics and such personal resources as health and cognitive status, and chronicity and severity of functional impairment. They also include an individual's preferences and expectations for specific characteristics of treatment programs. The environmental and personal systems influence each other through selection and allocation processes. For example, most programs select new patients on the basis of personal and psychiatric impairment criteria. Similarly, most

FIGURE 1.1.
A Model of the Relationships between Program and Personal Factors and Patients' Outcomes

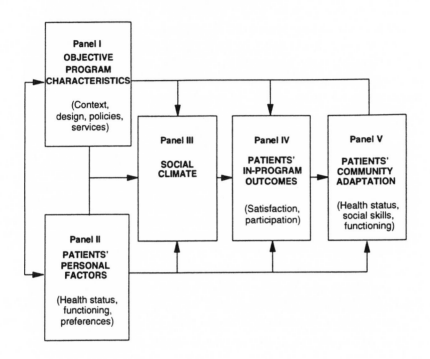

patients have some choice about the program they enter.

Both personal and environmental factors affect patients' in-program outcomes, such as their satisfaction, self-confidence, interpersonal behavior, and program participation (panel IV). In turn, in-program outcomes influence such indices of community adaptation as patients' health status, social and work skills, and psychosocial functioning (panel V). For example, on-site counseling and self-help groups and policies that enhance patients' decisionmaking (panel I) may contribute to a cohesive and self-directed social climate (panel III). In such a setting, a new patient may be more likely to develop supportive relationships with other patients and join a counseling group (panel IV) and, ultimately, to show better community adaptation (panel V).

The model shows that patients' adaptation is also affected directly by stable personal factors. For example, patients who have less severe symptoms when they enter a program are likely to have less severe symptoms a year later. Treatment programs may have some direct effects as well, as when an individual experiences better outcome because of the quality of treatment provided in a setting.

Finally, the model depicts the ongoing interplay between individuals and their treatment environment. Patients who voice a preference for more self-direction in their daily activities may help initiate more flexible policies (a change in the environmental system). Patients who participate more actively in psychotherapy or self-help groups may experience improved self-confidence (a change in the personal system). More generally, individual outcomes contribute to defining the environmental system; for example, when the in-program behavioral outcomes for all patients in a program are considered together, they constitute one aspect of the suprapersonal environment.

The model incorporates the characteristics of staff (panel I) and how staff influence the social climate and patients' in-program and community adaptation. We focus almost entirely on patients' outcomes here, but the basic model can be extended to encompass the health care work environment and it's influence on the treatment environment and staff members' morale and performance (Moos and Schaefer, 1987).

From a broader perspective, environmental factors external to the program profoundly affect patients' community adaptation. Hospital and community programs typically constitute only one time-limited aspect of patients' lives; accordingly, their influence may be short-lived. To understand the determinants of patients' psychosocial functioning in the community, we need to consider their family and work settings and their broader life circumstances (Moos, Finney, and Cronkite, 1990).

In the next sections, we describe two main lines of work that led us to focus on the characteristics of treatment programs: historical analyses and descriptive studies of how treatment environments alter patients' in-program symptoms and behavior, and comparative evaluations that illustrate how different programs affect patients' longer-term adaptation. In essence, this body of research suggests that characteristics of treatment programs, such as those included in panels I and III of figure 1.1, influence patients' in-program (panel IV) and community (panel V) outcomes.

Historical Background and Descriptive Studies

In modern times, the idea that treatment environments can change the patients and staff who live and work in them can be traced to Philippe Pinel, who in 1792 removed the chains and shackles from the inmates of two insane asylums in Paris. Most of the patients stopped being violent once they were free to move around. Pinel pointed out that people normally react to being restrained or tied with fear, anger, and an attempt to escape. Pinel applied "moral treatment," and assumed that the social or treatment environment, especially tolerant and accepting attitudes, setting examples of appropriate behavior, humanitarianism, and loving care, affects recovery from mental illness.

> I saw a great number of maniacs assembled together and submitted to a regular system of discipline. Their disorders presented an endless variety of character; but their . . . disorders were marshalled into order and harmony. I then discovered that insanity was curable in many instances by mildness of treatment and attention to the mind exclusively. . . . I saw with wonder the resources of nature when left to herself or skillfully assisted in her efforts. . . . Attention to these principles of moral treatment alone will frequently not only lay the foundation of, but complete, a cure; while neglect of them may exasperate each succeeding paroxysm, till, at length, the disease becomes established, continued in its form and incurable. (Pinel, 1806)

The Rise of Moral Treatment

In 1806 the Quaker William Tuke established the York Retreat in England, emphasizing an atmosphere of kindness and consideration, meaningful employment of time, regular exercise, a family environment, and the treatment of patients as guests. The Quakers brought moral treatment to America, and Charles Dickens (1842) noted the results in a lively account of his visit to the Institution of South Boston, later known as the Boston State Hospital.

> The State Hospital for the insane is admirably conducted on . . . enlightened principles of conciliation and kindness. . . . Every patient in this asylum sits down to dinner every day with a knife and fork . . . at every meal moral influence alone restrains the more violent among them from cutting the throats of the rest; but the effect of that influence is reduced to an absolute certainty and is found, even as a means of restraint, to say nothing of it as a means of cure, a hundred times more efficacious than all the straight-waistcoats, fetters and handcuffs, that ignorance, prejudice, and cruelty have manufactured since the creation of the world. . . . Every patient is as freely trusted with the tools of his trade as if he were a sane man. . . . For amusement, they walk, run, fish, paint, read and ride out to take the air in carriages

provided for the purpose. . . . The irritability which otherwise would be expended on their own flesh, clothes and furniture is dissipated in these pursuits. They are cheerful, tranquil and healthy. . . . Immense politeness and good breeding are observed throughout, they all take their tone from the doctor. . . . It is obvious that one great feature of this system is the inculcation and encouragement even among such unhappy persons, of a decent self-respect. (105–11)

Grob's (1966) history of the Worcester State Hospital in Massachusetts, which was established in 1830, documents the recognition of the importance of moral treatment and the patients' social environment (see also Kennard, 1983). He points out that Samuel Woodward, the first superintendent, thought that mental illness resulted from impaired sensory mechanisms: "If the physician could manipulate the environment he could thereby provide the patient with new and different stimuli. Thus older and undesirable patterns and associations would be broken or modified and new and more desirable ones substituted in their place" (53).

Woodward believed that mental illness was an outgrowth of detrimental social and cultural factors. The hospital implemented moral therapy, which consisted of a regular daily schedule and individualized care, including occupational therapy, physical exercise, religious services, and activities and games. Staff members were trained to treat patients with kindness and respect; physical violence and restraint were discouraged. The provision of moral treatment assumed that a healthy psychological environment could kindle renewed hope and cure individual patients. It implied that an appropriate social milieu could eliminate undesirable patient characteristics that had been acquired because of "improper living in an abnormal environment" (Grob, 1966, 66).

Although it is impossible to compare patients at Worcester in the 1830s and 1840s with patients today, the supportive structured climate of moral treatment may have been quite successful. Of more than 2,200 patients who were discharged from Worcester between 1833 and 1846, almost 1,200 or 54 percent were judged recovered. Moreover, in a long-term follow-up of almost 1,000 such recovered patients, in which information about the patient was obtained from family members, friends, employers, and clergy, nearly 58 percent were not readmitted to hospital and did not have a relapse (Grob, 1980).

Hospital Social Structure and Patients' Symptoms

The late nineteenth and early twentieth centuries witnessed a retreat from the principles of social treatment and increasing reliance on custodialism and physical restraint. During the 1950s and 1960s, however, theorists and clinicians again focused on the importance of the treatment environment. There was yet another reevaluation of the traditional disease model and its assumption that psychological disturbance resides in the individual alone. Hartmann's (1951) and Erikson's (1950) theoretical contributions reflected renewed interest in individual development and the link between external reality and perceptual and cognitive functions.

This focus was applied to try to understand the social structure and processes of psychiatric programs, which constitute the "reality" for hospitalized patients. Stanton and Schwartz (1954) and Caudill (1958) observed the importance of hospital social structure in facilitating or hindering treatment goals. Stanton and Schwartz's contribution revealed that patients' symptoms could be understood as a result of the informal organization of the hospital, that is, that the "environment may cause a symptom" (343). They found, for example, that hyperactive patients were typically the focus of disagreement between two staff members who themselves were seldom aware of this disagreement. The patient's hyperactivity often ceased abruptly when the staff members were able to discuss their disagreement.

Stanton and Schwartz also noted that a patient's dissociation may be quite reasonable in the face of certain social situations; for example, when two staff members strongly disagree about how to manage a patient, that patient may also be of a "divided mind." When staff disagreement or the "split in the social field" is resolved, the patient's dissociation usually subsides. Stanton and Schwartz (1954) conclude that "profound and dramatic changes such as observed in shock therapy . . . are no more profound and no more rapid than the changes produced . . . by bringing about a particular change in the patient's social field" (364). In addition, these authors showed how aspects of the hospital social environment, such as fiscal constraints stemming from financial pressure, may elicit staff conflict and confusion, which, in turn, generates low staff morale and collective disturbances among patients.

Caudill (1958) independently substantiated many of Stanton and

Schwartz's conclusions. In a clinical example, he revealed how the social structure of a psychiatric unit influenced a patient's behavior. Caudill showed how the patient's excited and disturbed behavior was due to his personal relationships with his therapist and with other patients. The therapist's interest in the patient was influenced by other staff members' attitudes, and the course of the patient's illness was closely associated with the hospital's therapeutic and administrative routines. Caudill (1958) concluded that "a patient's pattern of behavior cannot be sufficiently apprehended within the usual meaning of terms such as 'symptom' or 'defense,' but must also be conceptualized as an adaptation to the relatively circumscribed situation in which he is placed" (63). In another example, Stotland and Kobler (1965) show how a suicide epidemic in a hospital was directly related to changes in the hospital's financial and social structure and to resultant changes in staff morale, attitudes, and expectations of patient improvement.

Custodial Institutions

Although the development of moral treatment temporarily spawned a caring and humane social environment, as mental hospitals grew in size and complexity the emphasis on enlightened social treatment receded and institutions became more structured and custodial. The growing belief that immutable genetic and constitutional factors were the primary causes of mental illness contributed to this trend.

These changes led to the concept of "total institutions," which Goffman (1961) described as assuming absolute control over the life of people who reside in them. Total institutions break down barriers that ordinarily separate different domains of an individual's life, such as places of home, work, and recreation. In total institutions, all aspects of the residents' lives are conducted in the same place, that is, with a large group of other people who are all required to do the same things on a fixed schedule imposed by an apparently indifferent group of officials. Residents and staff interact with one another in restricted, formally prescribed ways. The rigidly structured, bureaucratic environment leads to apathy, passivity, and resignation among the residents.

Some hospital-based psychiatric programs in fact had many of the characteristics of a total institution. According to Wing and Brown (1970), who described Kerry ward, the ward door was always locked, and the patients lived almost entirely within the ward. There was little contact with the rest of the hospital and virtually no contact with the outside world. No patient went home, less than half were visited by relatives, and only a few were allowed to leave the ward without supervision. Movement about the ward was subject to close control. There were few if any exceptions to the restrictive policies. The hospital provided the patients' clothing, and few patients had any personal possessions on the ward or even owned a toothbrush. The lack of privacy was almost total. The lavatory doors did not lock, and baths were taken under nurses' and patients' direct supervision.

Patients were caught up in a daily routine that was geared to staff requirements. Staff did not encourage patients to develop personal skills; for example, staff made the patients' beds. In describing the daily routine on Kerry ward, Wing and Brown (1970) emphasize the paucity of social interactions and activities. They note that "there were long periods when most patients were simply waiting for the next stage of the cycle to begin; this waiting was mostly spent in apathetic inactivity, in doing absolutely nothing. All but 1 of the 22 patients in the series spent three hours a day sitting at a meal table and half were totally unoccupied except when eating or at toilet" (137). Such pervasive deprivation must have severe detrimental effects on patients, contributing to their stagnation and loss of hope.

Several well-known authors have compiled vivid and insightful case studies describing these widely divergent treatment environments and their impacts. Mary Jane Ward (1946) wrote of a custodial mental hospital's shocking physical and social environment and its detrimental effects in *The Snake Pit*. In Ken Kesey's (1962) *One Flew Over the Cuckoo's Nest,* patients respond adaptively to a rigidly structured ward setting that required them to submit to the authority of "Big Nurse." In sharp contrast, a warm supportive therapist and a constructive, humanitarian hospital facilitated a young schizophrenic girl's recovery in *I Never Promised You a Rose Garden* (Greenberg, 1964). In *The Magic Mountain* Thomas Mann (1952) vividly describes how the social environment of a tuberculosis sanitarium slowly and insidiously forces a patient to submit to its procedures and effectively give up his outside life and identity. Solzhenitsyn's (1969) *Cancer Ward* presents a similar tale, with a different outcome.

The Emergence of Community Care

Beginning in the 1940s in the aftermath of World War II, mental health reform began to focus on creating a normal environment for mentally ill individuals in the community in order to counteract the insidious effects of custodialism in large mental hospitals. Historically, these reforms were foreshadowed almost 100 years earlier in the Belgian city of Gheel, which developed a cottage-based moral treatment system in which mentally ill individuals lived in local family homes, worked alongside local villagers, and enjoyed considerable personal freedom.

Ironically, Merrick Bemis, the third superintendent of the Worcester State Hospital, proposed a decentralized, cottage-type reorganization of the hospital in the late 1860s (Morrissey and Goldman, 1980). According to Bemis's plan, most patients would live in small homes accommodating twelve to fifteen individuals supervised by a married couple. These homes would provide a family atmosphere, physical exercise and social activities, and supportive rehabilitative care. Although this proposal was never implemented, it captured some of the key ideas underlying the development of community-based therapeutic environments.

Reaction against custodialism grew in the 1950s, fueled by popular exposes and academic studies of the unacceptable conditions in mental hospitals and their detrimental effects (Belknap, 1956; Goffman, 1961). The National Mental Health Act of 1946 and the Community Mental Health Centers Act of 1963 provided the impetus for the development of community-based mental health programs, but also for the eventual transfer of responsibility for many patients from mental health settings to other systems, such as general hospitals and nursing homes (Brown, 1985; Mechanic and Rochefort, 1990).

Largely as a result of these reforms, the prevalence of inpatient care episodes in specialty mental health facilities in the United States declined from 77 percent in 1955 to 26 percent in 1990. In contrast, the prevalence of outpatient episodes rose from 23 percent to 67 percent. (Partial care accounted for 7 percent of the episodes in 1990.) Moreover, state mental hospitals accounted for 63 percent of the inpatient and residential treatment episodes in 1955 compared with only 16 percent in 1990. In contrast, such episodes in private psychiatric hospitals and non-Federal general hospitals rose from 30 percent in 1955 to 66 percent in 1990 (Redick et al., 1994). These changes are impressive; nevertheless, in part due to population growth, the total number of inpatient and residential care episodes in mental health facilities increased from 1.3 million in 1955 to 2.3 million in 1990.

It is difficult to obtain precise estimates of the number of clients and episodes of care in community residential facilities. Segal and Kotler (1989) estimated that between 300,000 and 400,000 chronically mentally ill individuals live in halfway houses, board-and-care homes, and other supervised community facilities. Similarly, Mor, Sherwood, and Gutkin (1986) identified 118 government programs for older adults that regulate more than 29,000 residential facilities with about 370,000 residents. In addition, between 30 and 75 percent of the 1.5 million patients in nursing homes may have serious psychiatric disorders (Linn and Stein, 1989).

Although these community facilities have not been rigorously studied, they encompass a wide variety of programs, including supportive, family-oriented programs, psychosocial rehabilitation programs, structured therapeutic community programs, and custodial programs. Thus, the treatment environments of community programs reflect the same diversity as those of hospital programs. Because residents may remain in community programs for extended intervals, it is especially important to study their treatment environments and outcomes.

Comparative Program Evaluations

Naturalistic and descriptive studies of hospital programs increased mental health professionals' awareness of the importance of the treatment environment, but they did not identify the precise characteristics that affect patients' morale, symptoms, and behavior. In the 1960s and 1970s, a number of investigators tried to isolate such characteristics by formulating treatment programs to achieve specific goals and then evaluating patients' reactions and outcomes.

Social Rehabilitation in a Therapeutic Community

In order to treat patients with personality disorders in a therapeutic community, Maxwell Jones (1953) founded the Social Rehabilitation Unit at Belmont Hospital in London, England. The emphasis was on communal life and the sharing of feelings to produce a meaningful experience in which individuals could grow and learn effective ways of functioning. The program was designed to involve patients in activities paralleling those of the community environments to which they would return. The unit incorporated group therapy, social activities, and work experience to provide patients with new social and job skills.

In an attempt to evaluate the rationale and effectiveness of this therapeutic community program, Rapaport (1960) considered the ideology, organization of patient and staff roles, and treatment and rehabilitation goals. The treatment ideology centered on the idea that "socioenvironmental influences are themselves capable of effectively changing individual patterns of social behavior" (269). The program employed paraprofessional staff to interact with patients, allowed staff roles to remain much less structured than in typical programs, and avoided restrictive rules and regulations.

Rapaport's study showed that the program was not as effective as its sponsors hoped. A major program purpose was to teach patients effective patterns of work and social behavior that could be generalized to their lives in the outside community. Staff tried to help patients become aware of the reasons for their behavior and to take an instrumental role in changing it. In addition, patients were required to assume some responsibility for the operation of the unit. Patients had a voice in this participatory democracy and became accustomed to determining their living and working environment. But the staff failed to recognize that most of the patients were from lower socioeconomic groups and were qualified only for unskilled or semiskilled positions, in which they would be heavily supervised and have few decisions to make. Self-understanding was not particularly valued. The treatment program had taught patients patterns of behavior that were basically inappropriate outside the hospital and thus could not generalize from the hospital to the community environment.

Problem-Oriented Task Groups in a Supportive Community

Fairweather (1964) constructed a different type of milieu program. He considered chronic mental patients as individuals who were capable of establishing roles and statuses in the hospital, but who were unable to do so in the community. The dependent role patients assumed in the hospital made it difficult for them to readjust to the community, where such a role is seldom available. Thus, Fairweather formed small problem-oriented task groups to provide chronic patients with experience in more active roles that could be transferred to the community at discharge. He structured a small group program characterized by autonomous task group meetings and compared it with a more traditional program.

Successful completion of the task group program involved four step levels of increasing responsibilities that entitled patients to more income and more liberal privileges. Task groups were responsible for orienting new members, evaluating members' performance, and making recommendations for job assignments, financial allotments, passes, and step level changes. The task group program emphasized involvement, autonomy, and program clarity and played down staff control. In contrast, patients in the traditional program were treated individually, and they requested help or privileges from the staff member assigned to work with them. Their role was much more passive and submissive.

Evaluations indicated that more patients in the task group preferred to be in a program other than their own; they felt that they had been deprived of leisure time and subjected to too much pressure to participate. However, the task group patients rated their unit more positively than the traditional unit patients rated theirs; they also believed that the unit had helped them more. They credited other patients for this help more frequently than they credited the staff.

A six-month follow-up showed that task group patients spent less time in the hospital, were more frequently employed, and were more actively involved with people outside the hospital. Nevertheless, 50 percent had returned to the hospital within the six-month period, suggesting that progress gained in the program was not necessarily maintained in the community. Why was this so? Fairweather reasoned that patients supported one another in the hospital, but they left the institution as individuals to enter the larger community, in which such support did not generally exist.

Following this line of thought, Fairweather and his colleagues (1969) established a community lodge and demonstrated that former mental patients could adjust to the community more effectively as a functioning task group than as individuals. The lodge program significantly increased employment and time in the community and enhanced members' self-esteem. More important, it cost only about half the amount of inpatient care. These findings show that individuals with chronic mental problems can adapt successfully in the community when they are in a supportive group and have active social roles. The lodge program has been widely adopted and replicated; it is an early model of the consumer-guided approach to community care.

Socioenvironmental Treatment and Expectations for Social Interchange

In a study of chronic schizophrenic patients, Sanders and his co-workers (1967) organized three comparable socioenvironmental treatment programs structured to vary the opportunity for social interaction. They thought that social interaction could be produced and enhanced by increasing the opportunity and demand for social functioning, and that the greater the external demand for interaction, the more favorable the outcome.

A minimally structured program offered patients the opportunity to interact, but staff did not exert any pressure. A partially structured program, which required patients to participate in teams that were responsible for housekeeping, included an interaction program with ten hours of group activities each week. A maximally structured program had the highest demand for interaction; it involved group therapy, individual work assignments, patient government, unit meetings, and so on. There was also a comparison group of patients who met the requirements for inclusion in the study but who remained in their original units.

The researchers analyzed improvement in terms of global social behavior and three social responses that reflected a hierarchy of social initiative: awareness of others, interaction in structured situations, and spontaneous social behavior. Socioenvironmental treatment improved some patients' social adjustment and psychiatric status, but exacerbated symptoms among other patients. The older men, and those with a longer duration of illness, showed the most favorable social response and the most positive psychiatric adjustment in the maximally structured treatment condition. The less structured treatment program also tended to benefit these men, but the effects were less marked. Traditional programs were entirely ineffective with such patients.

In contrast, younger men, and those with a shorter duration of illness, responded less favorably to socioenvironmental treatment. Some of these patients were disturbed by the interpersonal intimacy with members of both sexes that the treatment program required. Similar findings were not noted for women. A thirty-six-month follow-up indicated that, regardless of the degree of program structure, the effects of socioenvironmental treatment persisted in patients' posttreatment adjustment, although patients who experienced one of the two more structured programs tended to do better than those who participated in the minimally structured program.

A Social Learning Program

In an unusually well-designed study, Paul and Lentz (1977) focused on adult schizophrenic patients who had been hospitalized continuously for two years or more. These patients were randomly assigned to a skill-building social learning program, a milieu-oriented therapeutic community program, and a standard individualized supportive care program. All three programs included systematic aftercare services.

The social learning program emphasized patient-staff interaction, patient responsibility and problem solving, and a clear and well-organized structure. Patients were taught to display prosocial behavior and were rewarded when they did so; these rewards or tokens could then be used to obtain meals or privileges such as participation in desired activities. The emphasis was on skills training, with a focus on self-care, interpersonal communication skills, problem solving, stress management, and vocational training. There were also active attempts to generalize the skills training to less structured community environments and natural support systems.

The social learning program was the most effective and cost-efficient. More than 97 percent of the social learning patients were discharged from the hospital and remained in the community (typically in residential care facilities) for 90 days or more. This was true for 71 percent of the therapeutic community patients and only 45 percent of the supportive care patients. Moreover, social learning patients improved in all areas of functioning; almost 25 percent attained near normal levels in the specific skills targeted for change. The therapeutic community program also resulted in patients' improvement, but it had more problems, such as increased aggressive behavior, overstimulation of patients, and lack of generalization of skills.

In summary, each of the programs we have described followed a distinct theoretical rationale, and each accepted the basic idea that the treatment milieu has an important influence on treatment outcome.

Jones's program emphasized involvement, self-direction, self-understanding, and the open expression of feelings. Staff control was played down. Fairweather's program also encouraged involvement, and independence, but the main focus was on learning social and vocational skills rather than on self-understanding. Again, an attempt was made to minimize staff control. Sanders and his colleagues based their program on support and structure and, to a lesser extent, self-understanding and the open expression of feelings. Finally, Paul and Lentz focused primarily on patients learning specific self-care and social skills in the context of a highly structured program. Thus, we have four quite different programs; each claimed some success and each supports the idea that the treatment environment is related to patients' in-program and community outcomes.

Understanding Treatment Programs

Although clinicians and program evaluators recognized that the physical and social environment of psychiatric and substance abuse programs was influential, major questions remained unanswered. What program characteristics are related to different indices of in-program and community outcomes? Which characteristics have only short-term influences and which affect patients' longer-term adaptation in community? What type of program is best for what type of patient? To address these questions, it is necessary to systematically assess treatment programs and to document program implementation and compare alternative treatment settings.

Social Climate or the Perceived Treatment Environment

We focus most heavily here on social climate (panel III in figure 1.1). Much of the early research in this area involved naturalistic descriptions of psychiatric programs and other types of group living environments, such as correctional facilities, university students' residential facilities, and utopian communities (Moos, 1975, 1979; Moos and Brownstein, 1977). This work was valuable because it identified some key dimensions researchers could use to compare different types of settings, and it highlighted the connections between the social environment and individuals' mood and behavior.

In subsequent chapters, we describe the Ward Atmosphere Scale

(WAS) and the Community Oriented Programs Environment Scale (COPES), both of which are based on the social climate perspective. Each of these scales measures the quality of interpersonal relationships in a program, the emphasis on personal growth in specific areas, such as autonomy and the development of social and work skills, and the program structure.

Determinants of Treatment Environments

The WAS and COPES are based on participants' perceptions in that patients and staff members are asked to report on the characteristics of the treatment environment. As the work progressed, we turned our attention to four sets of factors that seem to be influential in shaping the social climate in treatment programs and in other types of settings:

- the institutional context, which encompasses such factors as for-profit or nonprofit ownership and a program's size and staffing;
- physical and architectural features, which can facilitate or impose constraints on the range of behavior in a program and influence specific patterns of patients' and staff members' activities;
- organizational factors, which include program policies such as how much choice patients have in their daily life and how much they participate in making decisions about program practices, and program services and social-recreational activities; and
- suprapersonal factors or the aggregate characteristics of the individuals in an environment, such as average age, gender composition, and cognitive impairment. These are situational variables in that they partially define relevant characteristics of the environment. This idea is based on Linton's (1945) suggestion that most of the social and cultural environment is transmitted by other people. It implies that the character of an environment is dependent in part on its members' typical characteristics.

Treatment Environments and Outcomes

Prior program evaluations and our own research on the variability of individual behavior in different contexts (Moos, 1968, 1969; Moos and MacIntosh, 1970) convinced us of the need to develop techniques to systematically characterize treatment environments. Naturalistic and empirical studies of psychiatric programs supported the belief that the treatment milieu was a key factor in understanding patients' outcomes. Accordingly, we examined the connections between hospital and community treatment programs and patients' in-program and community outcomes.

Overall, three sets of integrative concepts guided and grew out of this work:

- a framework of three underlying sets of dimensions that characterize social climates in diverse environments, such as psychiatric and substance abuse programs, the workplace, and task-oriented and mutual support groups;
- a conceptualization of four main sets of determinants of social climate; and
- a conceptual model to examine the processes that link the characteristics of patients and treatment programs and treatment outcomes, as shown in figure 1.1.

The Book in Brief

In chapter 1, we have presented a conceptual and historical overview and described the framework that guided and flowed from our research. Our work initially focused primarily on social climate, which is depicted as panel III in figure 1.1. Over time, we began to examine the institutional context, physical features, organizational indices, and suprapersonal factors that shape social climate (panel I in figure 1.1); in addition, we operationalized variables from the personal system (panel II), patients' in-program outcomes (panel IV), and patients' community adjustment (panel V).

The heart of the book is divided into three main parts. Part I focuses on hospital programs. In chapter 2, we describe the conceptual rationale and development of the Ward Atmosphere Scale (WAS) and the normative sample of 160 programs drawn from throughout the United States. We also focus on the diversity of treatment programs, patients' and staff members' preferences about treatment programs, and some psychometric and methodological issues. Chapter 3 focuses on how to monitor and improve hospital programs, and chapter 4 considers the assessment of program implementation.

Part II focuses on community programs. In chapter 5, we describe the Community Oriented Programs Environment Scale (COPES) and focus on the diversity of community treatment programs. Chapter 6 examines how to monitor and improve community programs, and chapter 7 focuses on the implementation of community programs.

The next four chapters, which comprise Part III, consider the determinants and outcomes of treatment environments. We discuss hospital and community programs together because we believe that common dynamic processes shape their treatment environments and patients' outcomes. Chapter 8 focuses on factors that shape the treatment environment. In chapter 9, we turn our attention to in-program outcomes such as patients' satisfaction and participation in program activities and, in chapter 10, we examine program factors associated with how long patients stay in the community and their adaptation and community living skills. Chapter 11 considers patient-program congruence and the apparent differential influence of treatment environments on patients who vary in their levels of impairment. This chapter also highlights the importance of the health care workplace and it's impact on staff and the treatment environment.

Chapter 12, which summarizes the findings, draws implications for program evaluation and design, and sets forth important issues for future research and practice.

Part I

Hospital Programs

2

The Social Climate of
Hospital Programs

More than 150 years after the emergence of moral treatment and the idea that a supportive and humane social environment can enhance patients' morale and well-being, we still know relatively little about the specific connections between treatment processes and treatment outcomes. In part, this is due to a lack of conceptually based measures of the quality of treatment. The program descriptions reviewed in chapter 1 highlight the diversity of hospital programs; however, they lack a common nomenclature and procedure for characterizing and comparing programs.

At the time we began our work in the 1960s, program evaluators were beginning to develop procedures to systematically assess psychiatric treatment programs. Thus, Jackson (1969) constructed the Characteristics of Treatment Environments scale to focus on program policies, such as the level of restrictiveness or freedom. Similarly, Ellsworth and his coworkers (1971) formulated the Perception of Ward Scales to assess such program factors as patients' concern for each other, emphasis on future planning, and communication among staff. As another example, King and Raynes (1968) developed the Inmate Management Scale to identify management- and patient-oriented program policies.

The Social Climate Perspective

We focus here on the development of a method to assess the social climate or treatment environment of hospital-based psychiatric and substance abuse programs. The social climate is the "personality" of a setting or environment, such as a treatment program, a workplace, or a family. In many ways, each environment has a unique "personality" that gives it unity and coherence. Like people, some social environments are friendlier and more supportive than others. Just as some people are self-directed and task oriented, some environments encourage self-direction and task orientation. Like people, environments differ in how restrictive and controlling they are. Individuals make plans to regulate and guide their behavior; likewise, environments have programs to regulate and guide the behavior of the individuals who live and work in them.

The concept of social climate and environmental demands or expectations has a long history. Murray (1938) noted that individuals have specific needs; the relative strength of these needs characterizes personality. To some extent, environmental demands can fulfill or frustrate these needs. Thus, Murray's model focuses on how the interplay between an individual's needs and an environment's demands influences the individual's cognition and behavior. Murray's concept of needs led to the development of new procedures to assess personality, but parallel development of measures of environmental demands has been much slower.

Stern (1970) noted that descriptions of environmental demands are based on inferred continuity and consistency in otherwise discrete events. For example, if patients in a treatment program are expected to talk openly about their personal problems, are asked personal questions by staff, are encouraged to share their feelings, and so on, then it is likely that the program emphasizes personal problem orientation, and, in turn, patients' self-disclosure and self-understanding. These conditions characterize one aspect of a program's social climate or treatment environment.

Our initial goal was to develop a standard method to measure the social climate or treatment environment of hospital-based psychiatric and substance abuse programs as appraised by patients and staff. Three principles helped to guide our work.

- Patients and staff members' perceptions provide an important perspective on a treatment program. Information about a program can be obtained from outside observers, who may be more "objective", but it is difficult for such people to know what the program is like without actually participating in it. Patients and staff members have time to form accurate, durable impressions of a program's treatment environment. Moreover, it is valuable to be able to compare patients' and staff members' views of a program.

- Program assessment is important in its own right. Many evaluators focus on outcome and assess only those aspects of treatment programs they think are related to the specific outcome they wish to explain. This approach can lead to the omission of factors that affect other outcomes and to superficial understanding of the program and the processes by which it functions. The salient aspects of treatment programs must be conceptualized clearly before we can evaluate their impact on patients' morale and behavior.

- The development of program assessment procedures should be guided by a flexible conceptual orientation. The idea of environmental demands or expectations helped us to formulate and select items that identify key characteristics of treatment programs. The framework of three sets of social climate factors shaped the organization of the dimensions to be evaluated. Prior work in this area lacked a conceptual framework and so produced isolated empirical findings that are difficult to organize into a coherent body of knowledge.

The Ward Atmosphere Scale—Real Form

Rationale and Development

We used several sources to obtain an initial pool of items for the Ward Atmosphere Scale (WAS). Two trained individuals with extensive experience in psychiatric programs observed three programs for several weeks, generating several hundred descriptive items. To identify characteristics of different types of psychiatric programs, we read several popular and professional books, such as Maxwell Jones's (1953) *The Therapeutic Community,* Ken Kesey's (1962) *One Flew Over the Cuckoo's Nest,* and Mary Jane Ward's (1946) *The Snake Pit.* We interviewed patients and staff who had been in different programs and asked them about these programs. These sources generated a pool of more than 500 items.

We then took three steps to develop an initial 206-item version of the WAS.

- We used Murray's (1938) and Stern's (1970) categories to select an initial set of twelve dimensions to describe treatment environments. According to two independent judges, twelve categories were adequate to cover the content areas identified in the item pool.
- We reduced item overlap in each of the twelve categories by deleting highly similar items. To control for acquiescence response set, we bal-

anced the number of positively and negatively worded items about equally within each category.

• We formulated twenty-three items to identify individuals who showed strong positive or negative halo in their perceptions. Some patients might agree with very positive items, such as "The food here is the best I've ever tasted" and "I never want to leave this program", whereas others might agree with very negative items, such as "In this program none of the staff members ever talk to any of the patients". These items also helped to identify inconsistent responses, because we could determine how often patients endorsed both very positive and very negative items.

The formulation of three underlying sets of environmental expectations or demands guided the choice and wording of specific items. More specifically, each item had to identify a program's emphasis on interpersonal relationships (such as involvement), on an area of personal growth (such as autonomy), or on organizational structure (such as order and organization). For example an emphasis on involvement is inferred from the following items: "Patients put a lot of energy into what they do around here"; "This is a lively program"; and "The patients are proud of this program." An emphasis on autonomy is inferred from these items: "Patients are expected to take leadership here"; "Patients here are encouraged to be independent"; and "Patients can leave the unit without saying where they are going."

An emphasis on personal problem orientation is inferred from still other items: "Patients tell each other about their personal problems"; "Personal problems are openly talked about"; and "Staff strongly encourage patients to talk about their past." Finally, an emphasis on order and organization is inferred from the following items: "Patients' activities are carefully planned"; "This is a very well organized program"; and "The staff make sure that the unit is always neat."

Construction of an Interim Form

We administered the initial 206-item form of the WAS to patients and staff in fourteen programs. These programs included three Department of Veterans Affairs (VA) programs for acute psychiatric and substance abuse patients, two VA programs for chronic psychiatric patients, two state hospital programs for chronically mentally ill patients referred from the criminal justice system, three state hospital programs for patients with acute and chronic psychiatric disorders, one private inpatient program for acute psychiatric patients, two psychiatric programs in community hospitals, and one program for acute patients on a university hospital teaching service.

Overall, 365 patients and 131 staff members in the fourteen programs responded to the WAS. To develop the interim version of the WAS, we tried to select items that discriminated significantly among programs and had no more than 80 percent of respondents answer them in one direction (either true or false). To control for acquiescence response set, we thought that each of the potential subscales should have a comparable number of items scored true and items scored false.

The use of these criteria resulted in a 130-item interim version of the WAS; that is, twelve content subscales each measured by ten items and a ten-item response set scale. One-way analyses of variance indicated that staff members' responses on all twelve subscales differentiated significantly among the fourteen programs; patients' responses on all but one subscale (involvement) differentiated significantly among the programs.

Psychometric Criteria and Final Form

The 130-item form of the WAS was administered to patients and staff in a normative sample composed of 160 psychiatric programs, in forty-four hospitals. These programs were located in sixteen states: Alabama, California, Colorado, Illinois, Kansas, Massachusetts, Mississippi, New York, North Carolina, Oklahoma, Oregon, Pennsylvania, Texas, Virginia, Washington, and Wisconsin. We included fifty-five programs in fourteen VA Medical Centers, fifty-five programs in ten state hospitals, twenty-eight programs in twenty-four university hospitals, and twenty-two programs in six community hospitals. A total of 3,575 patients and 1,958 staff members completed the WAS.

We used the data to develop the Real Form or Form R of the WAS. Because we did not then have the computer capability to analyze the entire sample at one time, we randomly sampled patients and staff from each of the 160 programs in proportion to their size. This process resulted in four subsamples, two of patients (Ns = 497 and 495) and two of staff (Ns = 437 and 439). In brief, the twelve *a-priori* subscales generally had excellent psychometric properties, except for the variety subscale, which we dropped due to low item intercorrelations and low item-subscale correlations. Because the involvement and affiliation subscales were highly intercorrelated, we collapsed them into one subscale labeled involvement.

To select items for the final form of the WAS, we applied five psychometric criteria:

- No more than 80 percent of respondents should answer an item in one direction (either true or false). This criterion eliminates items characteristic only of unusual treatment programs. Overall, 90 percent of the items met this criterion for patients or staff or both.
- Items should correlate more highly with their own subscale than with any other. All of the final items met this criterion.
- Each subscale should have a nearly equal number of items scored true or scored false to control for acquiescence response set. Of the seven ten-item subscales, two have five items scored true and five scored false; five subscales have six items scored true and four scored false. Two of the nine-item subscales have five items scored true and four scored false and one has four items scored true and five scored false.
- The subscales should have low to moderate intercorrelations. In fact, the average subscale intercorrelations are around .25, indicating that the subscales measure relatively distinct characteristics of treatment programs.
- Each subscale should discriminate significantly among treatment programs. All ten subscales met this criterion.

These scale construction procedures have contributed to the construct validity of the WAS subscales. Friis (1986a, 1986b) found that experienced psychiatrists tended to place the WAS items on their correct subscales. Moreover, an objective index of program autonomy was closely related to patients' and staff members' reports of WAS autonomy. In addition, O'Driscoll and Evans (1988) noted predictable associations between patients' and staff members' perceptions of a program's organizational structure and policies and the treatment milieu.

Table 2.1 lists the ten WAS Form R subscales and gives brief definitions of each. The complete WAS scoring key is in Appendix A. As shown in the table, the involvement, support, and spontaneity subscales measure relationship dimensions. The autonomy, practical orientation, personal problem orientation, and anger and aggression subscales tap personal growth dimensions. Order and organization, program clarity, and staff control assess system maintenance dimen-

TABLE 2.1
WAS Subscale and Dimensions Descriptions

Relationship Dimensions

1. Involvement   how active and energetic patients are in the program

2. Support   how much patients help and support each other; how
                              supportive the staff is toward patients

3. Spontaneity   how much the program encourages the open
                              expression of feelings by patients and staff

Personal Growth Dimensions

4. Autonomy   how self-sufficient and independent patients are in
                              making their own decisions

5. Practical Orientation   the extent to which patients learn practical skills and
                              are prepared for release from the program

6. Personal Problems   the extent to which patients seek to understand their
   Orientation   feelings and personal problems

7. Anger and Aggression   how much patients argue with other patients and
                              staff, become openly angry, and display other
                              aggressive behavior

System Maintenance Dimensions

8. Order and Organization   how important order and organization are in the
                              program

9. Program Clarity   the extent to which patients know what to expect in
                              their day-to-day routine and the explicitness of
                              program rules and procedures

10. Staff Control   the extent to which the staff use measures to keep
                              patients under necessary controls

FIGURE 2.1
**WAS Form R Means for Patients and Staff in 160 Programs
in the United States**

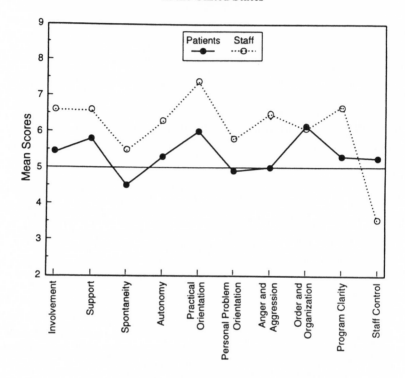

sions. These three underlying sets of social climate dimensions also characterize a range of other environments (Moos, 1994b).

The Diversity of Hospital Programs

Figure 2.1 plots the means of the Form R subscales for the 160 programs, separately for patients and staff. Staff report more emphasis than patients do in all areas except order and organization; they report less emphasis than patients do on staff control. As shown later, patients and staff in some programs agree quite closely. Nevertheless, these findings are consistent with the idea that staff members present a more positive picture of treatment programs that patients do, probably because they are responsible for organizing the programs and thus are more likely to understand them and to experience and emphasize their better aspects.

To better understand the specific areas in which patients and staff differed, we compared the two groups on each of the WAS items. Patient-staff differences were 20 percent or more on twenty-five items. For example, items on which staff answered true at least 20 percent more often than patients include: "Discussions here are very interesting"; "Staff are interested in following up patients once they leave the program"; "New treatment approaches are often tried in this program"; "In this program staff think it is healthy to argue"; and "Staff tell patients when they are getting better." Staff answered false more often than patients did on other items, including: "Once a schedule is arranged for a patient, the patient must follow it"; "Patients will be transferred from this program if they do not obey the rules"; "It is not safe for patients to discuss their personal problems around here"; and "Patients who argue with other patients will get into trouble with the staff."

Department of Veterans Affairs and State Hospital Programs

To learn whether there are broad differences in treatment programs in different types of hospitals, we divided the 160 programs into fifty-five from VA Medical Centers, fifty-five from state hospitals, twenty-eight from university hospitals, and twenty-two from community hospitals.

The fifty-five VA programs include programs for acute and programs for chronic patients, as well as programs primarily for psychiatric patients and those primarily for substance abuse patients. There were fifty-two programs for men, two programs for women, and one program for both women and men. The number of patients per program varied from twenty to 140, the number of full-time day staff from one to twenty, and the staff-patient ratio from 0.5 to more than 3.3 staff members for each ten patients. This part of the sample is composed of 1,687 patients and 590 staff.

The fifty-five state hospital programs include programs for acute and those for chronic psychiatric patients, programs for substance abuse patients, programs for youth, and programs with specialized treatment orientations such as cognitive behavioral and psychosocial rehabilitation. There are slightly more programs for men than for women. The

FIGURE 2.2
Patients' WAS Form R Means for Fifty-Five VA, Fifty-Five State, and Twenty-Eight University Hospital Programs

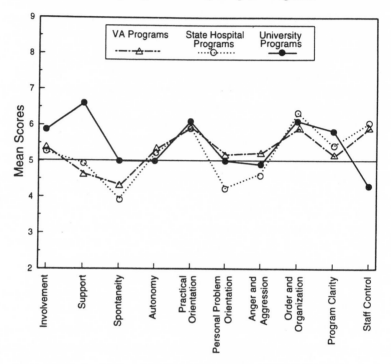

number of patients per program varied from seven to ninety; the number of full-time day staff from one to fourteen, and the staff-patient ratio from 0.3 to 5.7 staff members for each ten patients. The total number of patients and staff members in this part of the sample is 1,231 and 568, respectively.

Figure 2.2 compares patients' perceptions of VA and state hospital programs. On average, the two sets of programs are very similar, except that VA programs have somewhat more emphasis on personal problem orientation and the open expression of anger.

University Hospital Programs

Almost all the twenty-eight university programs were for both women and men. Many of these programs were composed of acutely disturbed patients. The number of patients per program varied from ten to forty, the number of full-time day staff from six to forty, and the staff-patient ratio from 3.3 to ten staff members for each ten patients. There were 391 patients and 532 staff members in this part of the sample. The number of staff members is high because trainees (such as psychiatric residents, psychology fellows, social work and nursing students) and evening and night shift staff were included.

According to figure 2.2, university programs have somewhat more emphasis on all three relationship dimensions and somewhat less emphasis on staff control than VA and state hospital programs do. Thus, university programs tend to involve patients more in treatment, to be more supportive, and to focus more on the open expression of feelings. They are less likely to restrict or try to keep patients under control. In part, these differences may reflect these programs' smaller size and more intensive staffing.

The results for the twenty-two community hospital programs are not plotted because of the limited sample. In brief, these programs were primarily for acutely disturbed short-stay patients. There were programs for women, for men, and for both women and men. The number of patients varied from ten to thirty; the number of full-time day staff from two to twenty-six, and the staff-patient ratio from 1.7 to ten staff members for each ten patients. This part of the sample includes a total of 266 patients and 268 staff members. Again, the number of staff members is high because trainee and evening and night shift staff were included.

Programs in the United Kingdom

To describe programs in the United Kingdom (UK) and examine the utility of the WAS for cross-cultural studies, we applied the WAS to a sample of thirty-six programs in the UK. The programs were drawn from eight hospitals and include three psychiatric programs in general medical hospitals, several programs in university teaching hospitals, and programs in both small and large hospitals in urban and rural areas. The median size of the programs was slightly more than twenty patients (range from seven to seventy-seven) and the median staffing was 2.5 full-time day staff members for each ten patients (range from less than 0.3 to more than nine). A total of 450 patients and 290 staff were included. (For more information about the norma-

FIGURE 2.3
**WAS Form R Means for Staff in Programs in the United States
and the United Kingdom**

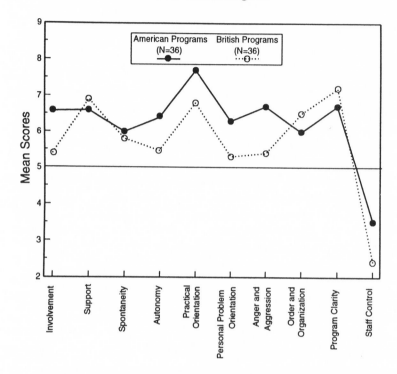

tive and psychometric characteristics of the UK sample, see Moos, 1972b, 1996b.)

To compare programs in the United States and the UK, we chose thirty-six programs from the American sample matched for the unit size and staffing ratios obtained in the UK. According to staff, programs in the United States are higher on involvement, on all four personal growth dimensions, and on staff control (figure 2.3). The differences for patients were comparable, although somewhat smaller (not shown).

Some items are especially sensitive to cross-cultural differences. For example, more American than UK patients and staff endorsed such items as: "Patients often do things together on the weekends"; "Patients are quite busy all of the time"; "Patients can leave the program whenever they want to"; "The staff act on patients' suggestions"; "Patients are expected to take leadership here"; "Patients who break the rules know what will happen to them"; and "Patients who break the rules are punished for it."

There is considerable overlap in the two samples; thus, some UK programs focus more on involvement, autonomy, self-understanding, and so on, than some American programs do. Consistent with a somewhat less prevalent psychosocial orientation, however, staff in the UK tend to develop less intensive programs that do not focus as strongly on expectations for patients' performance.

Psychometric and Methodologic Issues

We have examined the psychometric characteristics of the WAS and have focused on methodologic issues such as the search for factor dimensions and the effects of item context and respondent anonymity.

Internal Consistencies and Intercorrelations

We calculated internal consistencies and item-subscale correlations for each of the ten Form R subscales for patients and staff averaged over two random samples of twenty-three programs each. The internal consistencies were all in an acceptable range; they averaged .66 for patients and .71 for staff (see Moos, 1996b).

We intercorrelated the ten subscale scores for each of the four random samples. Very few of the correlations were as high as .40 to .50, accounting for only between 16 percent and 25 percent of the subscale variance (for the actual correlations, see Moos, 1996b). Thus, the ten subscales measure distinct but somewhat related aspects of hospital programs.

Halo and inconsistency response sets. As described earlier, we constructed an additional ten-item subscale composed of very positively or very negatively worded items to assess halo and inconsistency response sets (Moos and Houts, 1968). These items were endorsed by fewer than 10 percent of patients and staff and did not discriminate significantly among programs. We dropped this subscale from the WAS because the items in the ten content subscales were only minimally correlated with the halo and inconsistency scores; thus, these two response tendencies were essentially independent of the content subscales. In addition, because individuals who answer the WAS inconsistently or do not understand the items tend either not to complete the scale or to omit many items, these individuals' results typically are not included in characterizing a program.

Factor dimensions. Several investigators have identified a three-factor structure for the WAS, but the specific factors have varied (Alden, 1978a; Denny, Costello, and Cochran, 1984; Fischer, 1977). For example, Manderscheid, Koenig, and Silbergeld (1978) identified three factors that resembled the relationship, personal growth, and system maintenance domains (see also Friis, 1986a, 1986b). Squier (1994) found three somewhat related second-order factors labelled self-expression (high personal problem orientation and expression of anger), patient initiative (high autonomy and practical orientation, with low staff control), and organizational structure (high organization and clarity).

Although it is important to try to identify a small number of dimensions to characterize treatment environments, there are problems in looking for "the" factor structure of the WAS. Factor-analytic solutions are determined both by conceptual considerations and by aspects of the sample, statistical procedures, and criteria employed. More important, the proliferation of factor dimensions may impede the development of a consistent body of knowledge about the determinants and effects of conceptually meaningful aspects of treatment environments. (For more discussion of this issue, see Moos, 1990; 1994b.)

Reliability, Stability, and Differences among Programs

We calculated the test-retest reliability of subscale scores for forty-two patients, each of whom took the WAS twice one week apart. The results indicated that the ten subscales have adequate short-term test-retest reliabilities, which vary from .68 for practical orientation to .79 for involvement (Moos, 1996b).

We obtained profile stabilities by calculating intraclass correlations on the subscale standard scores of the different administrations of the WAS in a set of programs; these intraclass correlations reflect differences in both the level and relative position of subscale scores. The profile stability of programs that have a consistent treatment philosophy is very high over relatively long periods of time (Moos, 1996b). For example, in fifteen readministrations of the WAS over one-week to nine-month intervals, the average profile stabilities were .78 for patients and .86 for staff. In ten additional readministrations over fifteen-month to more than three-year intervals, the average stabilities were .75 and .86 for patients and staff, respectively.

The average profile stabilities over one- to three-year intervals are remarkable, because few if any of the same patients remained in these programs for six months or longer. Thus, the WAS measures aspects of the treatment environment that may remain stable despite a complete turnover in the population. As shown later, the WAS is also a sensitive measure of program change (chapter 3).

Kobos, Redmond, and Sterling (1982) similarly noted that the treatment environment of a psychiatric program maintained its stability despite rapid staff and total patient turnover in a six-month interval. Patients and staff in still another program showed stable perceptions of the treatment atmosphere on four occasions at six-week intervals in spite of considerable patient and staff turnover. The investigators thought that clear and explicit authority structure and open staff communication contributed to the stability (Schmidt, Wakefield, and Andersen, 1979).

The WAS subscales almost always discriminate significantly among programs for both patients and staff. We used Estimated Omega Squared to calculate the average proportion of the total subscale variance accounted for by differences among three sets of eight, twenty-eight, and thirty-six programs. On average, program differences accounted for about 20 to 25 percent of the subscale variance for patients and 25 to 30 percent of the variance for staff. Thus, a substantial part of the subscale variance is accounted for by differences among programs.

Respondent Anonymity

We conducted two studies in order to estimate the extent to which patients answer the WAS items differently depending on whether or not they put their names on the form. In the first study, patients in two programs were randomly placed into one of two groups, taken into separate rooms at the same time, and given the WAS under two conditions. In the first group, we gave the standard WAS instructions and told the patients: "Fill in your name in the space provided." We gave the patients in the second group the following instruction: "Don't bother to put your name on this scale. It is completely anonymous."

There were forty-nine patients in the name group and forty-five patients in the no-name group.

Means and standard deviations of each of the ten Form R subscales were obtained for each of the two groups and t-tests were computed between conditions. None of the ten subscales differentiated significantly between the name and the no-name groups. The two WAS profiles were essentially identical; the intraclass correlation between them was .80, and none of the standard scores for the two conditions differed from one another by more than one-half of a standard deviation.

The second study examined this issue under high threat conditions. Patients in the hospital in which the study was performed were legally committed and could be released only by staff consent. We expected these conditions to elicit maximum differences between name and no-name instructions.

Patients in each of four programs were randomly divided into two groups and assessed in the manner described earlier. One group of seventy patients was asked to put their names on the scale; another group of seventy patients was told that their responses were completely anonymous. Three of the subscales differentiated significantly between the two groups. Patients who put their names on the form reported more involvement and organization and less staff control. Thus, patients in the name condition viewed their programs somewhat more positively than patients in the no-name condition did. The two groups differed by about one-half of a standard deviation on the three subscales.

Under the usual low threat conditions of scale administration, therefore, it does not matter whether or not patients are asked to put their names on the form. In a potentially high threat situation, however, differences between name and no-name conditions may be as large as one-half of a standard deviation.

These conclusions hold only for patients. Because staff are more responsible for the treatment environment, they may be more likely to complete the WAS under conditions they perceive to be threatening; thus, staff may respond in a more positive direction than patients do. One way to minimize positive response distortion is to present the WAS items in a sealed booklet format (Makkai and McAllister, 1992; McAllister and Makkai, 1991).

Personal Characteristics and Program Perceptions

It is important to know how much individual demographic and personal characteristics affect perceptions of the environment. If these factors are strongly influential, perceived environment scales could be regarded simply as personality scales that happen to have items asking about the social milieu. In fact, most of the evidence is consistent with the conclusion that individual characteristics are only minimally associated with their perceptions of the treatment environment.

Demographic Characteristics

We first examined the extent to which individuals' gender, age, and length of stay (or time worked) in a program were associated with their perceptions of the treatment environment. For an initial sample of 365 patients in fourteen programs, only five of the thirty correlations were above .20 (Moos and Houts, 1968). Only two of the thirty correlations were above .20 in a second sample of 186 patients in eight other programs. The findings were similar for staff. Only eight of sixty correlations were above .20 in two samples of staff members.

Racial differences. According to Flaherty et al. (1981), African-American patients in one program reported poorer relationships and less emphasis on the personal growth dimensions than Caucasian patients did. African-American patients' negative appraisals may have occurred because they were given less responsibility and fewer privileges than Caucasians; or, their more negative perspective may have contributed to their being treated differently by predominately Caucasian professional staff.

Age differences. Compared with younger patients, older patients may be less well integrated into some treatment programs. In this vein, Linn (1978) found that older alcoholic patients reported less emphasis on personal problem orientation and the open expression of anger and more on staff control than younger patients did. Strasser, Falconer, and Martino-Saltzman (1992) obtained similar findings in a rehabilitation unit; in addition, older patients reported less emphasis on the relationship dimensions and on autonomy and practical orientation.

Overall, the associations between individuals' demographic characteristics and the WAS subscales are quite low. These results are consistent with findings in community programs (see chapter 5) and in other settings. For example, we identified only very modest associations between older adults' and staff members' personal characteristics and their perceptions of group living facilities (Lemke and Moos, 1987), few associations between residents' age and length of stay in correctional units and their perceptions of the unit's social environment (Moos, 1987), and close similarity between men and women residents' perceptions of coed dormitories (Moos, 1988). However, the findings for African-American patients and older patients described above suggest that individuals who are in a minority may perceive programs somewhat less positively than do those who are in the majority.

Personality and Role Factors

Social desirability. Patients and staff members who describe themselves in a socially desirable direction could also describe their program more positively. In contrast to this idea, however, we found few if any such associations for patients. In fact, patients with higher social desirability scores tended to see somewhat less emphasis on personal growth and somewhat more on system maintenance (Moos, 1996b). These findings imply that patients who describe themselves in more socially desirable ways may appraise their programs somewhat less positively.

We also examined this issue in a sample of staff members in four programs. Staff who answered items about themselves in a socially desirable direction had a slight tendency to answer the WAS items in a more desirable direction. The associations were generally low. Overall, patients' and staff members' tendencies to describe themselves in a socially desirable direction are only minimally if at all related to their perceptions of treatment programs. These results are consistent with those obtained on our other Social Climate Scales (Moos, 1975, 1979, 1994b).

Internal control orientation. Patients oriented toward an internal locus of control, who tend to be more striving, persistent, and self-confident than those who are oriented toward an external locus of control, may appraise their treatment programs as somewhat more supportive, higher on autonomy and practical orientation, and clearer and better organized (Baird, 1987; Greenberg, Obitz, and Kaye, 1978; Kish, Solberg, and Uecker, 1971a). These program characteristics may be congruent with internally oriented patients' expectations, which are to see the program as a locus of active treatment (see also Marone and Desiderato, 1982). Internally oriented patients may have more positive perceptions of programs because staff see them as having better prognoses and thus treat them in a more therapeutic fashion; externally oriented patients may be treated in a more custodial fashion.

Such processes can explain why patients' symptoms may be associated with their perceptions of a program. In this vein, compared to patients with more severe disorders, patients with less severe disorders evaluated their treatment programs as more supportive, practically oriented, clear, and well-organized (Vaglum et al., 1990). Compared with depressed patients, Baird (1987) found that nondepressed patients saw their program as more supportive, self-directed, and well-organized.

Staff roles and beliefs. Staff in more responsible positions in a program tend to view it more positively (Main, McBride, and Austin, 1991). Thus, Friedman, Jeger, and Slotnick (1980) assessed a program in which nurses had more responsibility for program functioning than other staff did. As expected, the nurses reported more involvement, support, and clarity and less staff control. Kish, Solberg, and Uecker (1971b) found that aides who held more conventional attitudes about treatment reported less program emphasis on autonomy and self-understanding whereas aides who believed that patients were accountable for their problems reported more emphasis on self-understanding (see also Zillmer, Archer, and Glidden, 1986). Compared to staff with a psychological treatment orientation, Squier (1994) noted that staff with a medical treatment orientation reported more organization and clarity and less self-understanding. Because each of these studies was conducted in several programs, however, the associations between staff beliefs and perceptions of the treatment environment may reflect in part actual differences among programs.

Overall, there are some associations between individuals' demographic and personal characteristics and their perceptions of the treatment environment, but such associations are seldom very substantial. Moreover, these associations may reflect important differences in individuals' experiences in a program. Patients with more severe disorders, or those who are in a minority, may be less well integrated into a program and thus appraise it less positively. Individuals' roles in a program also may affect their perceptions; specifically, staff members who are more responsible for and more active in a program are likely to see it more positively. As we describe later, patients' perceptions of a program may be associated with their long-term treatment outcome (chapter 10).

Patients' and Staff Members' Preferences

Clinicians and program evaluators have focused considerable attention on patients' ideas about optimal treatment programs. Not surprisingly, patients prefer supportive relationships with staff, individualized treatment content, availability of social and training activities, and participation in treatment decisions (Elzinga and Barlow, 1991; Hansson, Bjorkman, and Berglund, 1993; MacDonald, Sibbald, and Hoare, 1988). However, researchers have rarely considered staff members' value orientations about their treatment climate, and no available procedures tap patients' and staff members' values along the same dimensions. Moreover, we know of no procedures that enable evaluators to assess actual and preferred programs on common dimensions and thus to directly compare them.

The Ward Atmosphere Scale—Ideal Form

We developed the WAS Ideal Form (Form I) to enable patients and staff to describe the type of program they prefer; that is, to measure their goals and values about treatment programs. We wanted to identify areas in which patients and staff members have similar or different goals and to find out how much staff members' goals vary from program to program. We also wanted to compare actual and preferred programs and to give patients and staff an opportunity to identify areas they want to change.

The WAS Form I is parallel to Form R; that is, each of the items in Form I is parallel to one item in Form R. Form I can be used together with Form R to identify areas in which patients and staff want to change their program. Form I can also be used by itself to assess individuals' current preferences and to monitor changes in preferences among patients and staff.

An extensive sample of individuals in the United States and in the United Kingdom completed Form I. The sample of respondents from the United States consists of 2,364 patients and 897 staff from sixty-eight programs. The sample from the United Kingdom (UK) is based on 242 patients and 124 staff members from twenty-three programs.

Form I items and instructions and norms are provided in the WAS manual (Moos, 1996b).

Psychometric characteristics. We calculated item-subscale correlations and internal consistencies for the ten Form I subscales for a subsample of twenty programs (425 patients and 224 staff). The average item-subscale correlations varied from .33 for spontaneity to .51 for both personal problem orientation and anger and aggression. The subscale internal consistencies varied from .88 for spontaneity and order and organization to .71 for autonomy. Thus, Form I has adequate psychometric characteristics. In addition, individual preferences are quite stable over time; the average Form I profile stabilities for four programs assessed after intervals of six to twelve months were .78 for patients and .82 for staff.

Personal characteristics and preferences. There is some evidence that demographic and personal factors are related to staff preferences. Wolf (1978) noted that registered nurses who were better educated preferred more clarity, organization, and staff control and less autonomy and spontaneity. Nurses' length of work experience was not related to their preferences. Woods and Billig (1979) examined whether college students' vocational interests were related to their image of an ideal treatment setting. Compared with other students, those who wanted to become a physician, psychologist, or public administrator viewed an ideal program as providing more involvement and support and placing more emphasis on practical orientation and structure. These students' interest patterns were similar to those of physicians who were effective in treating psychiatric patients. Individuals who are interested in mental health careers may be more attuned to desirable aspects of treatment programs.

Preferences in the United States and the United Kingdom

American patients' and staff members' preferences are relatively similar, although staff prefer somewhat more emphasis on each of the relationship and personal growth dimensions and less on staff control (figure 2.4). These differences are comparable to those that exist in patients' and staff members' perceptions of actual programs (see figure 2.1).

Compared with patients in the UK, staff in the UK want more emphasis on all three relationship dimensions, all four personal growth dimensions, and program clarity, but less on staff control. Thus, the

FIGURE 2.4
WAS Form I Means for Patients and Staff in
Sixty-Eight Programs in the United States

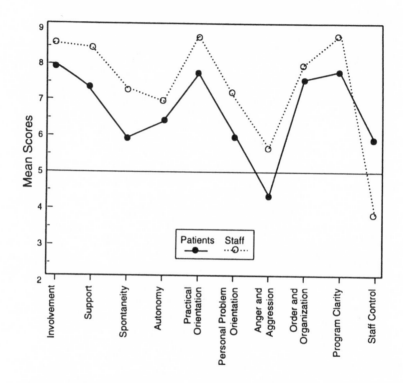

patient-staff differences are almost identical in the American and UK samples. These findings imply that staff members' roles and responsibilities shape loftier goals for ideal programs as well as more positive perceptions of actual programs.

We have described the rationale and development of the WAS, which assesses patients' and staff members' perceptions of the actual and preferred treatment environments of hospital-based psychiatric and substance abuse programs. The WAS has adequate psychometric properties, is quite stable over time, and can be used to compare programs in different sets of hospitals and programs in the United States and the United Kingdom. In the next two chapters, we turn to the use of the scale in monitoring and improving programs and in assessing the adequacy of program implementation.

3

Monitoring and Improving
Hospital Programs

Because of increasing concern about the quality and process of treatment, consultants and program evaluators are focusing more on carefully describing treatment programs and on systematically comparing programs with distinctive treatment orientations. In this vein, the WAS can be used to contrast patients' and staff members' views of the treatment environment, compare actual and preferred treatment climates, and provide feedback about the program to managers and staff. By monitoring changes in a program, it can also help to evaluate the impact of interventions and to plan and promote program improvement. These applications encourage staff involvement in program planning and design.

Describing Programs

We identified diverse WAS profiles in the normative sample; some examples of the more typical ones are given here. These descriptions focus on the program as a whole, analogous to the individual patient in a clinical case description. To facilitate direct comparisons, both patients' and staff members' scores are plotted in relation to patients' norms.

University Teaching Hospital Programs

Simon Ward is a heavily staffed, twenty-eight-bed, university service, acute treatment unit for women and men. There are between

FIGURE 3.1
WAS Form R Profiles for Patients and Staff on Simon Ward

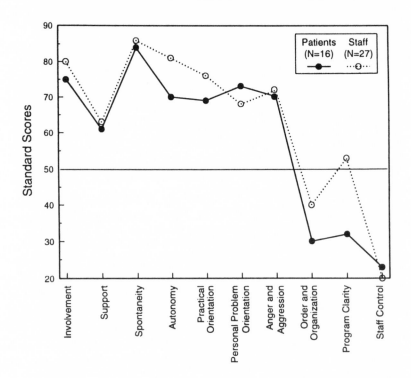

eighteen and twenty-six full-time patients, and between five and fifteen part-time patients. At the time of assessment, the staffing included the program director (a psychiatrist) and a psychologist; four psychiatric residents; three vocational rehabilitation counselors; two psychology trainees; and two part-time social workers. In addition, the program had a public health nurse, eight registered nurses, five licensed practical nurses, and seven psychiatric aides.

Figure 3.1 compares the WAS Form R profiles for patients and staff in this program with the average score obtained by patients in the American normative sample. There is striking agreement between patients and staff. Patients on Simon Ward are active and involved, spend time constructively, and are proud of the program. Performance expectations are high: patients are encouraged to be independent, to learn social and work skills, and to enhance their self-understanding

FIGURE 3.2
WAS Form R Profiles for Patients and Staff on Rulster Ward

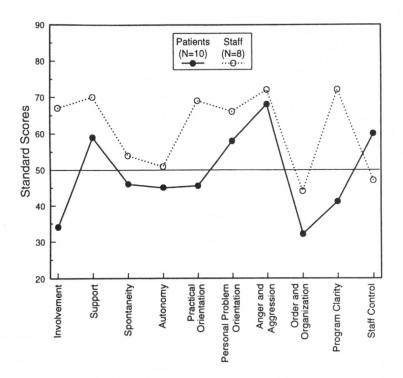

and express their anger openly. However, the program is not well structured; organization, clarity, and staff control are all below average.

The WAS findings are supported by other information about the treatment program. A patient first learns the community's basic expectations, which must be fulfilled if the patient is to earn necessities such as meals and a mattress. For example, lunch is earned by attending the morning activity that is part of a patient's individualized treatment program. To earn a mattress, a patient must hand in a personal daily program each evening. This behavioral approach contributes to the emphasis on practical orientation. Patients also obtain points by fulfilling personal treatment goals—for example, to become more involved with people, to increase self-confidence, to show and express feelings more openly. Such individualized goals contribute to the emphasis on personal problem orientation.

Simon Ward was reassessed after four months because staff wanted information about the stability of the treatment milieu. Even though all but one of the patients and most of the staff had changed, the profile remained essentially the same. The WAS profile stabilities were .92 for patients and .96 for staff, indicating very high stability over the four-month interval. Grant and Saslow (1971) discuss this program and highlight the value of obtaining regular assessments of treatment climate.

Figure 3.2 presents a contrasting profile for a different university teaching program—another small and heavily staffed unit. Rulster Ward had thirteen patients and eleven full-time staff members. The staff included a psychiatrist, a psychiatric resident, a psychologist, and several nurses and nursing assistants. Patients typically were acutely disturbed when admitted.

Although Simon Ward and Rulster Ward had quite similar structural characteristics and types of patients, their WAS profiles are quite different. Patients and staff on Rulster show moderate to high disagreement about the program. Both groups report above-average focus on support, self-understanding, and the open expression of anger, but staff see much more involvement, practical orientation, and clarity than patients do. Thus Rulster encourages patients to understand their feelings and express anger openly. According to patients, the program is moderately helpful and supportive; control is relatively strict.

Simon and Rulster Wards are both small psychiatric units located in university teaching centers. Both are highly staffed; both have relatively acute, short-term patients. However, the two programs have quite distinct treatment environments, which probably elicit quite different reactions from patients as they try to adapt to each program's expectations. On average, patients in Simon should be more satisfied and self-confident, be more likely to complete the program, and experience better adjustment in the community (see chapters 9 and 10).

A State Hospital Program

The next profile describes a program for men in a rural state psychiatric hospital. Sampson Ward is composed of forty-eight patients and seven full-time day staff members; some evening and night shift staff also completed the WAS. The program has several large, dormitory-type bedrooms and only minimally adequate physical facilities. Pa-

FIGURE 3.3
WAS Form R Profiles for Patients and Staff on Sampson Ward

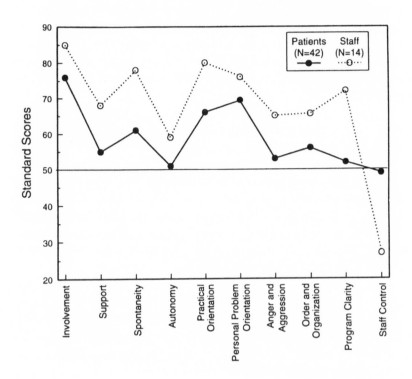

tients are subjected to relatively strict policies and there is very little privacy; however, there is an active patient government and a moderately intensive treatment program with several regular therapy groups.

Patients in Sampson Ward report above-average involvement and practical and personal problem orientation (figure 3.3). In addition, staff report strong emphasis on support, spontaneity, and the open expression of anger. Both groups agree that patients are somewhat encouraged to be independent; however, staff report much more focus than patients do on organization and clarity and much less on staff control.

Thus, patients and staff in Sampson Ward generally agree on the relationship and personal growth dimensions, although staff see more emphasis in these areas and a somewhat more differentiated program than patients do. In contrast, patients and staff disagree on the system

FIGURE 3.4
WAS Form R Profiles for Patients and Staff on Norman Ward

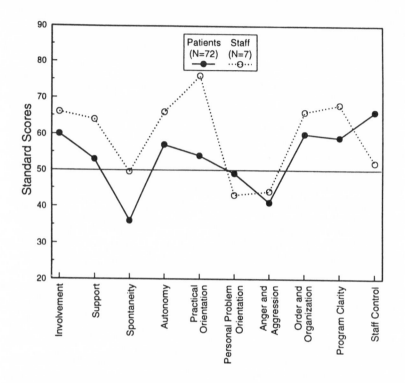

maintenance dimensions. We include this profile to show the type of treatment milieu that can be created with a difficult group of patients living in a relatively poor physical situation in a hospital with quite restrictive policies.

A Department of Veterans' Affairs Program

Figure 3.4 shows the WAS profile for a large program for eighty men in a VA hospital. The profile illustrates a relatively well-structured treatment environment. It shows that a relatively low staff-patient ratio—about one staff member for every ten patients—does not necessarily result in unclear expectations or a disorganized program.

Patients and staff in Norman Ward report a high level of organization, clear program rules and procedures, and a moderate level of staff control. Patients are asked to keep their behavior within clearly defined limits. Patients and staff also report above average involvement, autonomy, and practical orientation, but staff see more focus on each of these areas than patients do. However, both groups agree that the program does not encourage self-understanding or the open expression of anger.

Thus Norman Ward is a quite large, not particularly well-staffed VA hospital program in which all three system maintenance dimensions are seen as important. The relatively large size and low staffing may necessitate a high level of structure to keep the program functioning adequately. In addition, the program emphasizes some aspects of the relationship and personal growth dimensions, most notably involvement, autonomy, and the development of social and work skills. The profile indicates that large size and minimal staffing do not necessarily preclude the development of a coherent treatment environment.

Actual and Preferred Treatment Environments

A more detailed picture of a program can be drawn when patients and staff members provide information about both the actual program and their preferences. Lathrop Unit is a small VA program with between twenty and twenty-five male patients and seven full-time day staff members. Patients saw the program as emphasizing independence and self-direction, but as close to average on all nine of the other WAS dimensions. In contrast, staff reported above average emphasis on support and spontaneity, on all four personal growth dimensions, and on organization and clarity.

Figure 3.5 compares the amount of change patients and staff want in the program, as indexed by subtracting the average subscale score for the actual program from the average score for an ideal program. For the program to become an ideal program in the eyes of patients and staff, each area would have to increase or decrease as shown in the profile. The line in the center of the profile indicates that no change is desired; that is, that there is no discrepancy between the actual and preferred environment. For example, staff want no change in autonomy or staff control. Positive scores indicate a wish for more emphasis, whereas negative scores reveal a desire for less.

As shown in Figure 3.5, patients and staff want more emphasis on each of the relationship dimensions and on the development of social

FIGURE 3.5
Real-Ideal Discrepancies as Seen by Patients and Staff on Lathrop Unit

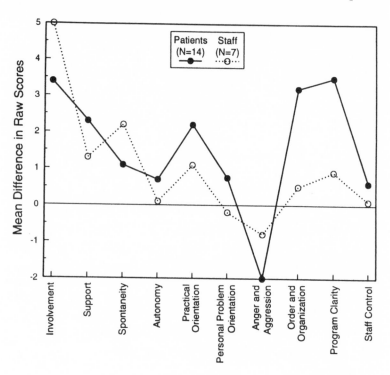

and work skills. Staff are relatively satisfied with organization and clarity, but patients want much more focus on both areas. Both groups want less emphasis on the open expression of anger. As we describe later, this information has implications for changing the program. Patients and staff can discuss their views of the program and can try to alter it in line with their preferences.

These profile descriptions indicate that the WAS can highlight the distinctive characteristics of a treatment environment, help to understand a program's potential problem areas, and compare programs with each other. We turn next to applications of the scale in monitoring program change, teaching staff about program characteristics, and helping staff improve programs.

Monitoring Program Change

In addition to describing treatment programs, the WAS can be used to monitor the process of change in existing programs and to guide the development of new programs. Substantial changes may occur when a program's overall treatment orientation is altered, as reported by Schmidt, Wakefield, and Andersen (1979) and Verhaest (1983). When implemented adequately, most program modifications eventually result in greater involvement, support, and expressiveness. Changes in the personal growth dimensions are linked somewhat more to the specific kind of program change that takes place. Thus, Ng, Tam, and Luk (1982) noted that the addition of nondirective community meetings in an inpatient program helped to promote a climate of spontaneity and self-disclosure, and several investigations recorded increases in practical orientation in social learning or behavior modification programs (Eriksen, 1987; Gripp and Magaro, 1971; Willer, 1977).

On the other hand, many program modifications do not stimulate either large or long-term changes in the treatment milieu. Specific but delimited policy changes such as granting patients the right of access to their hospital records (McFarlane, Bowman, and MacInnes, 1980), banning smoking (Smith and Grant, 1989; Thorward and Birnbaum, 1989), or rotating physician interns (Sparr et al., 1994) typically fail to produce major changes in a treatment milieu.

Social Learning Programs

In general, the development of programs based on social learning or behavior modification principles tends to enhance practical orientation and autonomy, as well as involvement; however, clarity sometimes declines temporarily. Eriksen (1987) restructured a short-term inpatient alcoholism unit into patient and staff teams and developed a new program based on social learning principles. Patients and staff reported increased practical orientation and autonomy; involvement, organization, and clarity also rose. Some social learning principles were also initiated in a halfway house program, which showed comparable but smaller changes than those in the inpatient program.

To evaluate the development of a social learning program, Gripp and Magaro (1971) compared the experimental unit with three nonintervention units. Nursing staff completed the WAS prior to initiating the new program and again six months later. According to staff, the social learning program became more task focused and oriented toward autonomy, as well as more involving and expressive. Unexpectedly, organization and staff control declined, perhaps because staff initially had problems understanding how to apply social learning principles. There were no consistent changes in the nonintervention programs. Patients in the social learning program improved more than did those in the comparison programs. Moreover, staff in the social learning program rated it as more congenial and therapeutic and reported a greater sense of responsibility, accomplishment, and morale.

Schmidt, Wakefield, and Andersen (1979) studied a day-care program in which they introduced goal-setting groups, patient contracts, and a patient government. Patients and staff completed the WAS prior to the changes, shortly after the changes were made, and several months later. Immediately after the changes, patients and staff described more acceptance of the open expression of anger but also less clarity. Several months later, both groups reported more support and self-direction; they also saw the program as better organized, clearer, and less controlled by staff (Schmidt et al., 1980). Thus, the program changes created a situation in which patients felt more independent and responsible (see also Curtiss, 1976).

Individualized Patient Programming

In individualized programs, case managers work with patients to set specific, individualized goals and provide patients with personalized feedback and evaluation as embodied in a goal-oriented record system. Willer (1977) evaluated the implementation of such a program in an inpatient unit of a psychiatric hospital; a comparable unit in the same hospital served as a no-treatment comparison. Patients in the individualized program reported increases in autonomy and practical orientation; staff reported improvement in these two areas, in the open expression of anger, and in organization. Moreover, patients in the individualized program showed better community adjustment, and male patients showed lower rehospitalization rates.

The development of standard assessment procedures and new targeted treatment modules can also improve a treatment program. In one substance abuse program, a host of problems arose from low staff morale, conflicts within the nursing staff, lack of communication between staff members, inadequate assessment of patients, inability to provide effective rehabilitation, and misunderstanding of higher-level managers. After securing help from the hospital administration and conducting an initial assessment, Lacoursiere and Bradshaw (1983) held weekly meetings of a reorganization planning committee, developed new staff assessment teams, and implemented several new treatment modules. Staff members were apprehensive at first, but the continued change effort eventually succeeded. After nine months, staff attitudes had markedly improved and the new treatment program was judged to be superior to the old one.

Designing a Therapeutic Community

When custodial or medically oriented programs are reoriented toward therapeutic community (TC) principles, the quality of relationships usually improves and the emphasis on autonomy, self-understanding, and the open expression of anger increases. Ingstad and Gotestam (1979) monitored the change in the treatment milieu of a psychiatric unit that shifted from primarily custodial practices to a more active TC orientation. Patients and staff completed the WAS before the program reorientation and again six months later. Staff reported increases in all relationship and personal growth dimensions, but felt that the program was less well organized. Patients reported more support, self-direction, and practical orientation.

To monitor the maturation of a TC, Verhaest (1983) administered a Dutch translation of the WAS four times over a six-year interval. The initial changes focused on improving interpersonal relationships and promoting autonomy; involvement and the expression of anger rose and the level of staff control declined. However, staff learned that they had to set limits and restrain freedom for severely disturbed patients; accordingly, autonomy and the expression of anger declined and there was a rise in staff control. The focus on limit setting and structure eventually led to a further evolution of the TC emphasizing reality confrontation, sharing of decision making, and active exploration of personal problems. Support and expressiveness remained high, and autonomy and practical orientation increased. In this example, the WAS helped to track ongoing program changes and to identify the extent to which the intended treatment ideology was realized.

Models of Stepped Versus Continuous Care

Some treatment programs use a stepped model of care in which new patients are placed into an admission unit and then, after the acute phase of their illness subsides, are transferred to a predischarge unit. The stepped model separates acutely ill from less disturbed patients and enables staff to work with more homogeneous patient groups. In contrast, a continuous care model in which patients are treated in one unit from admission to discharge has the advantage of offering patients continuity of care and of giving staff the opportunity to follow patients' progress throughout their hospital stay.

In an evaluation of these alternative systems of care, Long, Blackwell, and Midgley (1990, 1992) compared a continuous care unit with admission and predischarge units in a two-stepped system of care. Staff in an admission unit that became a continuous care unit reported an increase in spontaneity and the open expression of anger; however, organization declined. Patients in the continuous care unit reported more spontaneity and practical orientation; unexpectedly, they saw the program as less involving and supportive as well as less organized. It may have been more difficult to establish a supportive and structured climate in the continuous care unit because patients' tended to stay in the program for a much shorter interval than did patients in the stepped unit system.

Compared with predischarge unit staff, staff on the continuous care unit saw it as placing more emphasis on the development of social and work skills and on self-understanding. Compared with predischarge unit patients, however, patients in the continuous care program saw it as less involving, self-directed, and organized, perhaps because of their shorter hospital stay.

The introduction of the continuous care unit enhanced staff morale and performance. Compared with admissions and predischarge staff, nursing staff on the continuous care unit reported more job satisfaction and less uncertainty about treatment procedures, made better use of their skills and abilities, and were absent less often. Compared with admission unit nurses, continuous care nurses also demonstrated better problem-solving skills and communication with nursing peers. Overall, caring for a more varied group of patients under the continuous care model seemed to enhance staff morale, but a shorter hospital stay may diminish this model's potential positive effects on the treatment environment and patients' long-term adjustment. (For a project in which acute care units were transformed into admission units, see Leiberich et al., 1993.)

Staff Education and Models of Care

Several studies have shown that staff education in specific models of care can improve the treatment environment in predictable ways. For example, Stirling and Reid (1992) evaluated a program in which nurses learned a participatory control model of patient care that emphasized clear communication, problem solving, setting specific goals, and understanding and interpreting patients' behavior. Patients cared for by nurses who learned this model reported increases in autonomy and spontaneity on the unit, and a decline in staff control. In addition, patients developed a more positive self-concept and showed an increase in their self-perception of control. No such changes were shown by an attention control or a no-contact comparison group.

To measure the implementation of a human needs model of nursing, McKenna (1993) administered the WAS in two long-stay psychiatric units before the introduction of the model, midway through a nine-month implementation period, and at the end of nine months. At first, there were no differences in the treatment milieu between the intervention and a comparison program. After the introduction of the human needs model, patients and staff in the intervention program reported improvements in the treatment environment; no such changes occurred in the comparison program. After nine months, the human needs model program was more supportive and oriented toward patients' personal growth than the comparison program was. Nursing care plans also were of better quality and patients were more self-directed and satisfied and less dependent.

Staff involvement in intensive training in inpatient group therapy can substantially improve a treatment program. According to Leviege (1970), there were large post-training differences between a program on which staff received intensive training that emphasized self-understanding and actual practice in encounter group techniques and a program in which staff had no group therapy training. Patients and staff described the intervention program as more involving, expressive, and oriented toward self-direction and self-understanding. They also thought that it was better organized and less controlled by staff. Staff in an-

other program were provided with informal training in group techniques; patients and staff in this program saw the treatment environment somewhat more positively than patients and staff in the control
program did, but not as positively as did patients and staff in the
intensive intervention program.

Staff Members Wearing Uniforms or Regular Clothes

Some clinicians believe that the quality of patient-staff relationships
will improve if staff members wear regular clothes rather than uniforms. To test this idea, Klein and his colleagues (1972) organized a
three-stage project in which staff members wore traditional uniforms,
changed to wearing street clothes, and then returned to wearing uniforms. They assessed attitudes toward and perceptions of self, others,
and the program during each stage. There was an initial three-week
baseline (stage one), followed by a six-week period (stage two) during
which nursing staff wore street clothes. During the last three-week
period (stage three) the nursing staff returned to wearing traditional
uniforms. The study was conducted on a twenty-eight-bed, heavily
staffed, milieu-oriented unit in a university hospital.

Klein and his colleagues found that the treatment environment remained basically stable regardless of changes in nursing staff dress.
Contrary to expectations, however, patients felt somewhat more se-
cure and less anxious, rated themselves and other patients as less
distant, and saw themselves as better models for their own behavior
when nursing staff wore uniforms. They also had more confidence in
the staff and rated them as emotionally healthier, more supportive, and
easier to identify.

Staff also found the change to and from street clothes to be disruptive; moreover, they experienced disappointment and an apparent loss
of self-esteem when required to return to wearing uniforms. Staff members rated nursing staff as most difficult to identify at stage two, when
they were wearing street clothes, and they perceived the treatment
environment as less clear at that time. There was less involvement and
interpersonal support and more disruption in the program during stage
three; however, these changes were most likely related to a turnover in
residents and staff at that time. The evaluators concluded that there
was no clear evidence that wearing street clothes facilitated closer
therapeutic engagement between staff and patients. It is possible, how-

ever, that the comparatively short interval of stage two (six weeks) and the subsequent need for nurses to revert to wearing uniforms precluded any larger or more permanent change.

Program Relocation

Because programs are often moved from one part of a hospital to another, it is important to examine the impact of intrahospital relocation. Kelly (1983) asked staff members to assess the social climate of open and closed units for chronic psychiatric patients before and after a relocation. Staff who moved from one closed unit to another rated the new program as more supportive, well organized, and task oriented and as lower on staff control. Staff who moved from one open unit to another saw no differences in the treatment environments. As expected from these findings, the relocation did not have a detrimental effect on patient functioning. The positive outcome probably was caused by continuity of care in a familiar environment and by an ongoing schedule of supportive activities in the overall hospital setting.

In another relocation study, the WAS showed no changes in the treatment environment of a psychiatric and an alcohol treatment program that were relocated. However, the relocation of these two units had a negative impact on an adjacent psychiatric unit that did not move; there was a decline in involvement and support (Flaherty et al., 1980). Finally, Hills (1987) noted that relocation can cause differential changes in the treatment milieu, depending on the types of patients relocated and associated changes in the physical features of the unit and in staff.

Promoting Program Improvement

Program evaluators can use information about the treatment milieu to enhance program development. Here we describe the use of the WAS as a teaching aid and as a way to facilitate staff discussion and program change. (For other studies in which the WAS has helped to improve treatment environments, see Friedman, 1982; Friedman, Jeger, and Slotnick, 1982; Kish, 1971; Verinis and Flaherty, 1978.)

The WAS as a Teaching Aid

The WAS can be used to educate staff about their program's treatment environment and how to change it. In this vein, patients and staff in a small, heavily staffed university teaching program completed the WAS on four occasions over a two-year interval. Patients initially reported somewhat below average emphasis on involvement and on all four personal growth dimensions. The staff basically agreed with the patients, but they reported more personal problem orientation and open expression of anger and less staff control than the patients did.

After a consultant gave the staff feedback on this profile, staff members decided to try to develop a structured therapeutic community program. The consultant's use of the WAS as a teaching aid followed a four-step approach. First, the consultant presented the WAS results for the current program and discussed patients' and staff members' profiles as compared to the norms. When patients and staff disagreed by more than one standard deviation, the subscales were discussed item by item to find out why.

In the second step, actual and preferred profiles were compared. Areas in which there were large discrepancies were analyzed and the specific items on the relevant subscales were discussed in detail. During this process, staff members sometimes changed their preferences. Staff members of different roles often disagreed sharply. For example, compared with nurses, the program director and psychiatric residents wanted more emphasis on involvement and expressiveness and less on staff control.

After intensive discussion, the third step involved an attempt to formulate a common goal—for example, an increase in involvement and autonomy. The items from these subscales were then placed on the staff bulletin board. At first, staff enacted the behaviors reflected in the items somewhat automatically and without appropriate affect; within a few weeks, however, patients and staff began to assimilate the spirit of the items.

The results of a reassessment several months later, which constituted the fourth step in the change process, indicated that the program had developed a more active treatment environment. Patients and staff saw much more emphasis on involvement and on all four personal growth dimensions than they had initially. The basic thrust of the program was to emphasize self-direction, self-understanding, and the development of patients' social and work skills. The substantial changes in these areas brought the program much closer to an ideal program as envisioned by both patients and staff. Most important, the overall improvement in this program's treatment climate shows that assessment and intensive staff discussion can promote positive change.

Facilitating Change by Feedback and Staff Discussion

We conducted another project to improve a psychiatric program in an urban general hospital. Damien Unit serves twenty-five women and men both as full-time inpatients and day patients. It is an acute, short-term program and has a major commitment to training mental health professionals, including psychiatric residents, psychology and medical interns, and psychiatric social work fellows. Because of the training commitment, the staff-patient ratio is high, about 1 to 1.5 staff members per patient on the day shift. The initial treatment orientation was psychodynamic; individual and group psychotherapy were major treatment components. The patients participated in community meetings that focused primarily on program policies, scheduling activities, and the introduction of new patients and staff (Pierce, Trickett, and Moos, 1972).

The staff decided to use the WAS to describe the treatment milieu and to plan and evaluate changes in the program. The first WAS profile, shown in figure 3.6, indicates that neither patients nor staff saw much emphasis on the relationship or personal growth dimensions. In fact, both groups reported below average involvement, autonomy, and practical orientation. Both groups also saw organization and staff control as below average.

Providing feedback and planning change. A consultant presented the WAS profiles to the staff in feedback sessions. Staff comments focused on autonomy and staff control, reflecting a concern about patients' lack of progress. The program did not promote patients' autonomy; staff did not exert sufficient influence on patients, who were too dependent and comfortable. This problem was especially evident in the lack of progress of a group of patients who had been in the program for a relatively long time. Another issue involved managing those aspects of patients' impulsive behavior that were clearly beyond program rules and required staff to set limits.

At the end of the feedback sessions, staff completed the Real Form

FIGURE 3.6
Initial WAS Form R Profiles for Patients and Staff in Damien Unit

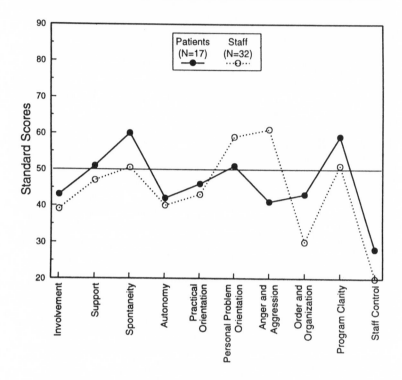

of the WAS again to reassess the program before any major changes were introduced and to evaluate the stability of the program over a five-month period. Two weeks later staff completed the Ideal Form.

As an outgrowth of the discussions in the feedback sessions a staff committee was formed to generate suggestions and to reorganize the community meetings. Another staff committee reviewed the activity program and offered ideas to increase patients' and staff members' participation in program activities. The treatment team meetings focused on patients whose length of stay exceeded the average expectation for the program and on improving staff members' consistency in setting limits on patients' impulsive behavior.

Several changes were initiated as a result of the committee reports and the new focus in the treatment team meetings. Staff became much more active in structuring community meetings, specifically by clari-

FIGURE 3.7
Follow-Up WAS Form R Profiles for Patients and Staff in Damien Unit

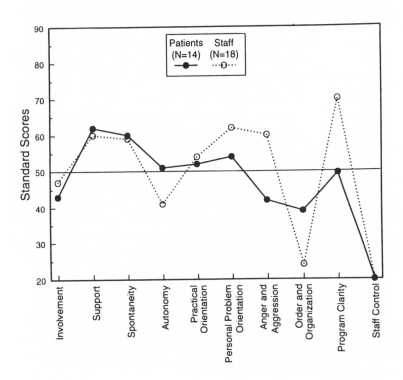

fying their expectations of patients and discussing program norms and values. The treatment team assumed responsibility for managing patients' impulsive behavior and all staff agreed to abide by the team's decisions. To enhance the continuity of care and the consistency of treatment, staff actively encouraged patients' outside therapists to attend meetings and participate in program decisionmaking. Eight months after the initial assessment, patients and staff completed the WAS again to identify changes that had occurred in the interim.

Program improvement. Figure 3.7 shows the follow-up profiles for patients and staff. A comparison of figures 3.6 and 3.7 indicates that staff reported more emphasis on support and spontaneity as well as on practical orientation and clarity. Patients saw a more supportive program that focused more on self-direction and the development of social and work skills. These changes reflect a more differentiated treatment program that is much more in line with staff preferences. The overall shape of the profile remained relatively stable, reflecting the fact that the changes took place gradually, within a consistent treatment philosophy.

We reviewed the medical records of several patients whose progress became an area of focus during the project. The records revealed increased staff activity and increased patient movement. Some patients were discharged to day-care and other after-care programs; other patients were transferred from full-time to day patient status. Overall, there was more rapid patient turnover.

Changes in staff preferences. Staff completed the WAS Form I again eight months later. During this interval, the program shifted from a psychodynamic model to a model that emphasized crisis intervention, short-term treatment, and resocialization within the context of the therapeutic community. Staff became more concerned with patients' interpersonal and social functioning, the control and regulation of patients' behavior, encouragement of independence, and hospitalization as a temporary resolution to crisis.

Cooper (1973) theorized that these changes would predictably influence staff members' preferences. He correctly hypothesized that preferences for personal problem orientation, the open expression of anger, and staff control would decline. These changes reflected a deemphasis on intrapsychic processes and self-understanding, a de-emphasis on patients being submissive and cared for by staff, and more focus on patients' control of impulses such as the expression of anger.

Cooper's prediction that staff preferences for spontaneity and autonomy would rise were less well supported in that these preferences changed only slightly. Cooper speculated that the emphasis on impulse control and on patients working together in groups may have raised staff members' concerns about group controls and made them less willing to promote autonomy and spontaneity. Overall, however, the changing nature of the program predictably influenced staff members' preferences.

Improving Inpatient and Day Hospital Programs

In an alcohol rehabilitation program in which there was a sudden increase in irregular discharges, the WAS showed a concurrent decline in support, spontaneity, practical orientation, and clarity (Verinis, 1983).

After staff became aware of these changes, the program regained a more therapeutic atmosphere with significant increases in patients' reports of autonomy, organization, and clarity; the proportion of irregular discharges declined to its former level. By providing feedback to staff that the treatment milieu was not functioning effectively, the WAS helped to restore it to its original therapeutic condition. (For an example in a Danish program, see Ejsing, 1980.)

Herrera and Lawson (1987) focused on a clinical research unit that had low staff morale and a high level of violence and injuries to patients and staff. The WAS results were used to understand the unit's milieu and to develop goals. Readministered three months later, the WAS showed significant improvement in staff perceptions of the program, greater patient-staff agreement, and a lower level of patients' aggressive behavior and staff's use of seclusion and restraint.

Changing a day hospital program. Milne (1986) used the WAS to identify problems and to evaluate the implementation of subsequent changes in a day hospital program. Nurses and patients held similarly unfavorable views of the program at two baseline assessments; they reported low levels of involvement, support, spontaneity, and clarity. This finding helped in planning systematic changes that led to augmented staff training in behavior therapy and anxiety management and to regrouping patients into acute and chronic groups that were treated on different days.

The acute patients felt that the program improved, as did the staff with respect to the days on which the acute patients were treated. In contrast, the chronic patients saw the program as somewhat worse, as did the staff on the days the chronic patients were treated. In essence, the chronic patients served as a comparison group, because the program changes were directed primarily toward the acute patients. A follow-up showed that the acute patients improved during treatment, whereas the chronic patients showed some deterioration. According to Milne (1988), the organizational changes produced better treatment outcome and showed that the WAS has "treatment validity" because it enabled a consultant to improve a treatment program.

Problems in forming a therapeutic community. Ongoing feedback about the treatment environment can facilitate changes in a program, but the resulting improvement may not survive broader structural changes in a hospital. In this vein, Friis (1981a) conducted a six-year longitudinal study using a Norwegian version of the WAS to monitor a psychiatric program and promote its development as a therapeutic community (TC). This process moved ahead only after a host of problems were overcome, including recruiting staff, differentiating the TC from other programs in the hospital, and obtaining sufficient autonomy to develop the program as a TC (Friis et al., 1982). After the treatment climate improved, administrative problems in the hospital forced the program to become a closed unit primarily for acute psychotic patients. Subsequently, the treatment environment returned to roughly what it had been prior to the intervention.

These projects raise a question about the effectiveness of specific procedures consultants use to provide feedback to staff. To examine this issue, James, Milne, and Firth (1990) gave one group of staff written feedback only, while a second group also had four monthly meetings to discuss the feedback and plan strategies for reducing real-ideal program discrepancies. The WAS was readministered during the course of the four-month intervention and again six weeks after it was completed. The feedback contributed to changes in several program procedures and to a reduction in real-ideal discrepancies in the system maintenance dimensions. This effect was greater for staff who had the opportunity to discuss the feedback and plan changes.

Change-Oriented Teaching and Evaluation

As the preceding examples show, the WAS can be used to assess and change treatment programs. Giving patients and staff feedback about the treatment environment guides them to focus on difficult or problematic aspects of the program. It helps them to understand that they can alter the program and to plan specific changes to do so. (For other examples of action research projects to change hospital programs, see Barker and Barker, 1994; Boyd, Luetje, and Eckert, 1992; and Lavender, 1987.)

By measuring a program's treatment milieu, giving feedback, and planning interventions, program evaluators and consultants can:

- encourage patients and staff to think about their program along the ten dimensions of the WAS instead of in an oversimplified way such as "good" or "bad," and "stressful" or "not stressful";
- highlight important but often overlooked program characteristics, such as the clarity of expectations and the level of patient autonomy;
- focus patients' and staff members' efforts to improve their program on

a few well-defined areas so as to reduce confusion and increase the likelihood of orderly change; and
- provide an opportunity for program directors and staff to consider their impact on the treatment environment and on patients.

Importantly, providing information about the treatment program can help to promote ongoing teaching and program evaluation. By initially tying teaching or evaluation to current issues in a program, staff can help plan and participate in informative and important projects. As Carroll et al. (1980) have shown, an active research program can provide an impetus to improved treatment. In this regard, busy staff who lack extensive facilities or personnel for evaluation can use easily administered assessment procedures such as the WAS to quickly obtain information about their program's functioning.

We have shown that the WAS can be applied to describe a broad range of psychiatric and substance abuse programs in the United States and in other countries. Moreover, the scale can help to monitor the development of innovative programs, such as social learning and therapeutic community programs, and to promote program change. We turn next to the use of the scale in assessing program implementation and comparing programs.

4

Assessing the Implementation
of Hospital Programs

No treatment is so direct or obvious that an evaluator can take its implementation for granted. Accordingly, an assessment of how treatment is actually implemented is an integral aspect of developing innovative treatment approaches and evaluating treatment outcome. Yeaton and Sechrest (1981) recommend that an assessment of treatment implementation should include both the program's strength "the a priori likelihood that the treatment could have the intended outcome" (156)—and its integrity—"the degree to which treatment is delivered as intended" (160).

Many programs are ineffective because they are not adequately implemented; an implementation check helps researchers avoid evaluating a poor example of the intended intervention. An assessment of treatment strength and integrity makes it possible to gauge prognosis on the basis of information about treatment as well as information about patients. It highlights logical fallacies in the standard pessimistic interpretation of intervention program evaluations. For example, a few sessions of outpatient treatment may have a short-term positive influence on a client, but they probably are not strong enough to exert a measurable impact several years later.

Assessing treatment implementation is the first step in understanding the content of treatment and in carefully studying the treatment process itself. Here we discuss several methods and criteria for assessing treatment implementation. Then we describe implementation assessments of a range of programs, including acute admission and rehabilitation programs, substance abuse programs, therapeutic community programs, and an intentional social systems treatment model.

Assessing Program Implementation

To find out how well a program is implemented, an evaluator must measure the actual program against a standard of what the program should be. Sechrest and his colleagues (1979) identified three sources of information that can be used to define a standard for program implementation: normative data on conditions in other programs, which allow the evaluator to see how one program compares with others; specifications of an ideal treatment program; and theoretical analyses or expert judgment. In chapter 3 we provided examples of the normative approach in comparing several hospital programs to the WAS normative sample (figures 3.1 to 3.4), and of the specification of an ideal program as seen by patients and staff (figure 3.5).

From a broader perspective, it is important to measure both the quantity and quality of program activity in an assessment of treatment implementation. The quantity of treatment is indexed by each patient's treatment experiences, such as the number of individual and group psychotherapy sessions attended, the intensity of vocational rehabilitation services received, and so on. In this vein, participation in specific components of treatment and the length of treatment tend to be associated with better treatment outcome (McLellan et al., 1994; Moos et al., 1990; Moos et al., 1995b). Whereas information on treatment components reflects the quantity of treatment activities, treatment "quality" refers to the manner in which such activities are carried out. We use the WAS as one way to measure the quality of a program's treatment environment.

Acute Admission and Rehabilitation Programs

One basic implementation question is whether programs with contrasting treatment goals and orientations actually develop different treatment climates. Compared with three acute admissions programs, Cruser (1995) noted that two resocialization programs emphasized vocational training and paid employment, and patient-staff cooperation to schedule activities and maintain order. Consistent with these differences, resocialization staff saw their programs as more supportive, well orga-

nized, and practically oriented. However, resocialization patients reported only more organization. Thus, compared with their goals and
the admissions programs, the resocialization programs were well implemented according to staff but not according to patients.

The resocialization programs did not fare well according to normative standards. Patients and staff reported below average support and
only average involvement and practical orientation. Cruser (1995) highlights the value of this type of information for program planners and
staff.

In a comparison of five VA programs, Kish (1971) noted that one
program used a social-psychological approach, a second was oriented
more traditionally toward medications and activities, and a third, an
alcoholism treatment program, used an educational approach centered
on Alcoholics Anonymous (AA). In the other two programs, treatment
depended more on individual staff members' preferences and judgments; no attempt was made to develop an official treatment philosophy. The areas of emphasis in the first three programs generally were
consistent with their stated treatment orientations indicating that the
programs were well-implemented. For example, patients and staff in
the alcoholism program saw the milieu as high on involvement and
practical and personal problem orientation. These qualities are consistent with a program emphasizing participation in AA, group therapy to
promote self-understanding, and social and vocational rehabilitation.

Unexpectedly, patients and staff reported considerable emphasis on
order and neatness in the program that was oriented toward social-
psychological treatment. This finding raised concern that the program
was too structured and eventually led to an examination of transactions made through notes, which were the main method for communication between the treatment team and the patient groups. When it was
revealed that 30 percent to 50 percent of the notes were concerned
with such matters as unmade beds and dusty lockers, staff tried to
lessen the emphasis on order. Staff members also formulated specific
programmatic changes to reduce the disparities between their own and
patients' perceptions of the treatment milieu. Kish notes that program
evaluators can provide a useful service for treatment teams by admin-
istering scales such as the WAS and providing feedback about the
adequacy of program implementation.

There has been considerable interest in the development of specialized programs for Vietnam veterans with posttraumatic stress disor-

ders. In one such program, an evening component incorporated an active vocational rehabilitation and work reentry orientation. Patients viewed this program as oriented toward the development of work and social skills; they also saw it as supportive and expressive, oriented toward self-understanding, and clear and well organized (Pendorf, 1990). Practical orientation and staff control were somewhat higher in the evening than in the regular day program. These findings show that the overall program was adequately implemented and that an emphasis on work and job training can be effectively incorporated into an evening program.

To develop a biopsychosocial rehabilitation model for the treatment of chronic psychiatric patients, Burda and colleagues (1991) formulated an integrated program incorporating a broad range of therapeutic interventions. Patients saw this program as high on the relationship dimensions, oriented toward autonomy, and clear and well organized. Follow-up data showed high patient satisfaction and a positive impact of this well-implemented program on patients' functioning.

Sometimes local administrators think that programs in which staff members profess common treatment orientations actually have similar treatment milieus. When Pullen and Clark (1983) assessed seven apparently comparable inpatient units in a psychiatric rehabilitation service oriented toward social treatment, however, the WAS showed considerable variation among them. Feedback of the findings clarified that each program actually had a treatment environment that was appropriate for its residents' needs. Several other researchers have used the WAS in this way to check the implementation of treatment programs for schizophrenic patients (Bernstein, Heim, and Ballinari, 1983; Glick and Hargreaves, 1979; Stanton et al., 1984).

Substance Abuse Programs

In an assessment of Satori, a structured therapeutic community for substance abuse patients, Moffett (1984) found that the treatment environment was consistent with program principles: relatively high on the relationship and personal growth dimensions and well organized with clear and explicit rules. Satori's focus on control was expressed through a program structure in which patients' impulsive behavior was minimized by extensive rules that were enforced mainly by the patients themselves. Several years later, Satori was described as highly

FIGURE 4.1
WAS Form R Profiles for Patients and Staff in Peer Confrontation Program

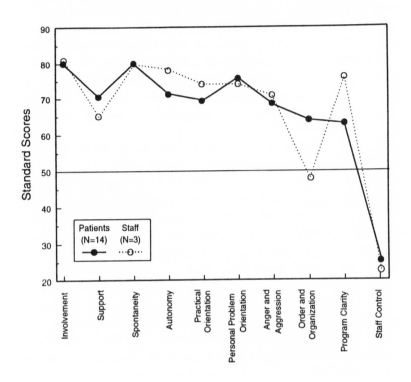

involved and spontaneous, task-focused, oriented toward self-disclosure and the open expression of anger, and clear and relatively well
organized. Satori's social climate was distinctive, stable, and consistent with its intended design as a therapeutic community for personal-
ity-disordered, substance dependent men (Moffett and Flagg, 1993).

One idea, stimulated partly by Synanon, is to have patients assume
substantial responsibility for organizing a substance abuse program
and for confronting each other's problems and dysfunctional behavior.
Van Stone and Gilbert (1972) described one such program, which was
housed on an open unit and was composed of thirty men who sought
help primarily because of substance abuse. Each patient negotiated an
individualized contract with his peers describing his goals for behavior
change. In addition, each patient was confronted candidly in the peer

therapy group about any self-defeating or dishonest behavior. The patients controlled the program and made decisions about each patient's level of responsibility, status, and duties in the program.

The program had only three regular staff members and, thus, was minimally staffed according to the usual criteria. Even so, patients and staff agreed closely in appraising the program as unusually well implemented (figure 4.1). Both groups saw a high level of involvement and support and considerable emphasis on self-direction, skills training, self-understanding, and the open expression of anger. They also saw the program as clear and well organized. The majority of patients who stayed in the program for two weeks or more improved; patients who stayed in the program longer tended to improve more.

Therapeutic Communities

Several studies have focused on the implementation of therapeutic community (TC) programs. Verhaest, Pierloot, and Janssens (1982) compared two TC programs with different treatment orientations. One program emphasized psychodynamic psychotherapy; the other was more structured and oriented toward teaching and education. As expected, the more structured program was higher on practical orientation, organization, and staff control, whereas the psychodynamic community was higher on autonomy. However, there also were some surprises; the structured community was more involving and oriented toward self-understanding. Verhaest and his colleagues (1982) described how these unexpected findings helped to understand and change the programs.

In another comparison, Lehman and his colleagues (1982) studied first-admission patients in a TC program or a traditional, medically oriented psychiatric program. The TC program was higher on involvement, autonomy, practical orientation, and the open expression of anger; the medically oriented program was better organized. These differences were predictably related to specific treatment process differences, such as more use of family treatment in the TC program. Patients and staff in the TC program were more satisfied, but there were no significant differences in two-year program outcomes.

The findings were similar in another comparison of a TC and a medically oriented program. Patients and staff in the TC program saw it as higher on autonomy and the open expression of anger; staff also saw the TC program as more involving and spontaneous. In contrast, the medically oriented program was higher on practical orientation and better organized (Trauer, Bouras, and Watson, 1987). The WAS profiles suggested that the medically oriented program was better implemented: compared to the TC program, patients and staff in the medical program agreed more closely about the treatment milieu and the program profile was much more stable over time. In fact, the TC program became more like the medical program, suggesting that complex and atypical programs have a tendency to revert to become more like prevalent ones. Trauer et al., (1987) speculate that it may be especially difficult to maintain a TC program in a medically oriented psychiatric environment (see also Friis, 1981a).

Therapeutic communities in short-stay programs. A few studies have been conducted to ascertain whether TC principles can be implemented in short-stay inpatient programs. Steiner, Haldipur, and Stack (1982) evaluated six acute admission units in a community mental health center, three of which supposedly were organized as TCs. The WAS showed no differences between the three apparent TCs and the other three programs; moreover, the TCs did not conform to the empirically derived TC program profile (Price and Moos, 1975).

The Street Ward Community at Fulbourn Hospital, Cambridge, is an acute admission unit that tries to function like a TC, even though the average length of stay for a resident is fewer than seventeen days. Staff saw the atmosphere as high on autonomy, self-understanding, and the open expression of anger and as lacking in organization. In contrast to the findings of Steiner et al. (1982), these results imply that a TC can be established within a short-stay acute psychiatric admission program (Pullen, 1982; see also Lindsay, 1986; Pullen, 1986). Compared with short-term admission units, however, longer-term treatment programs tend to be more involving and oriented toward patients' personal growth (Squier, 1994).

Therapeutic communities in forensic hospitals. A related question is whether it is possible to implement a TC in a maximum security forensic hospital, given the conflicting institutional goals of treatment and control. According to Caplan (1993), patients saw one such program as both supportive and controlled. Staff saw the program as more involving, organized, and clear than patients did. Reflecting the structured nature of the program, both patients and staff reported little emphasis on spontaneity or the open expression of anger. Thus, this program was well implemented with respect to support and structure, but not with respect to the expression of affect or the other personal growth areas.

Medical Programs

A number of investigators have applied the WAS to assess the implementation of medical programs, including oncology units, dialysis units, and rehabilitation programs.

Oncology units. According to Alexy (1981–82), patients, staff, and family members differed in their perceptions of the actual and preferred treatment climate of an oncology unit for adolescents and young adults. Patients wanted much clearer information about what to expect in the day-to-day routine of the unit. Staff saw the need for clarity but also wanted the program to be more supportive and organized. Family members were especially concerned about the need to emphasize self-understanding and for staff to exercise more control over the youthful patients. Such information can help to identify patients' and family members' concerns, as well as those of staff, and to suggest ways to improve implementation of medical programs.

Dialysis programs. Patients and staff in a chronic hemodialysis program reported a similar emphasis on the relationship and system maintenance dimensions, but staff saw more focus on patients' social and work skills, self-understanding, and the open expression of anger (Rhodes, 1981). As sometimes happens in psychiatric programs (Baird, 1987), depressed patients saw the program somewhat more negatively than nondepressed patients did, perhaps because they were not as well integrated into it. Alternatively, depressed patients may focus on the dysfunctional aspects of their environment and filter out positive features to maintain a negative perceptual set.

An adapted version of the WAS has been applied to patients and staff in seven Israeli dialysis programs (De-Nour, 1983). In general, patients and staff members saw the programs quite differently, indicating important variations in program implementation. Consistent with the findings in psychiatric programs, staff tended to see more emphasis in most areas than patients did. Patients in a more involving and supportive program seemed to be more satisfied and better adjusted.

Rehabilitation programs. Strasser and his coworkers (1994) focused on three interdisciplinary rehabilitation health care teams in one hospital. Unexpectedly, the three teams tended to see the "same" hospital environment differently on nine of the ten WAS subscales. The teams also differed in their group climate, as assessed by the Group Environment Scale (GES; Moos, 1994a). The team that saw the hospital environment as least supportive, clear, and, self-directed was itself the lowest on cohesion, organization, independence, and task-orientation. These findings imply that variations in a team's niche in the overall hospital setting may affect the team's functioning. Alternatively, how well rehabilitation teams function may color their members' perceptions of the broader hospital milieu. (For another application to a rehabilitation program, see Strasser et al., 1992.)

In another study, an adapted version of the WAS was used to compare patients who participated in a team-oriented rehabilitation program with patients who did not. Perhaps because they were more actively included in treatment, the patients in the team-oriented program reported more support from staff and other patients, more concern about their personal problems and feelings, and less staff effort to maintain control (Crisler and Settles, 1979).

Children's Programs

The WAS has been used to assess the implementation of psychiatric inpatient programs for children (Wolff et al. 1972), to compare residents' and staff members' views of a residential center for developmentally disabled adolescents (McGee and Woods, 1978), and to examine the treatment environment of a residential center for emotionally disturbed children and youth (Feist, Slowiak, and Colligan, 1985). Staff in the residential center saw the treatment milieu as supportive and tolerant of anger and as well organized and clear, perhaps at the expense of promoting independence and responsibility. Clients generally agreed with staff, but they saw much less emphasis on the relationship dimensions and on organization.

Steiner (1982) applied the WAS to an inpatient psychosomatic unit for children and adolescents. These young patients described the program as a therapeutic community, which shows that an active treatment milieu can be implemented in the context of conjoint intensive psychiatric and medical treatment of patients with psychosomatic disorders. Compared to a pediatric unit, the psychosomatic unit was more structured and had more emphasis on self-understanding and the open expression of anger. The pediatric unit had a cohesive social milieu with relatively high involvement, support, and spontaneity (Terry et al., 1984).

In a reassessment of the psychosomatic unit ten years later, Steiner, Marx, and Walton (1991) found high stability in both patient and staff perceptions even though there was complete turnover in patients and more than 60 percent turnover in staff. The treatment environment was still quite similar to that in a structured therapeutic community. In addition, there was a "maturation effect" in that patient-staff agreement rose. Thus, a treatment environment can remain adequately implemented despite many changes in the health care system, especially a shorter length of patient stay, higher patient acuity, and nursing staff shortages and turnover.

A Typology of Hospital Programs

By identifying general types of treatment programs, an evaluator can develop more specific standards against which to assess the implementation of new programs. Thus, as we saw earlier, Steiner et al. (1982) compared the WAS profile for a short-stay admission unit with our empirically developed therapeutic community profile to assess the implementation of TC principles. To enhance this use of the WAS, we conducted a cluster analysis of WAS data based on patients' perceptions of 144 programs and identified six types of treatment programs: therapeutic community, relationship oriented, action oriented, insight oriented, control oriented, and undifferentiated (Price and Moos, 1975). These six types closely resemble the types found in community treatment programs (see chapter 7).

Therapeutic Community and Relationship-Oriented Programs

We identified nineteen programs as a therapeutic community cluster. As shown in figure 4.2, they are well above average on relationship and personal growth dimensions, but low on system maintenance dimensions. Patients are active and involved and are encouraged to express their feelings freely, to be independent, to learn social and work skills, and to discuss their personal problems. The programs are somewhat lacking in structure, probably because of staff members' concerns about restricting patients' freedom. These programs tend to be located in university teaching hospitals and to be small and highly staffed.

FIGURE 4.2
**WAS Form R Profiles for Patients in Therapeutic Community
and Relationship-Oriented Programs**

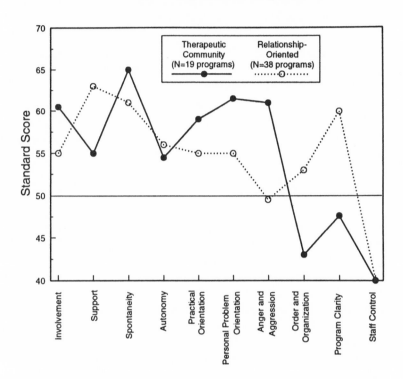

Figure 4.2 also profiles the thirty-eight programs identified as relationship oriented. These programs are well above average in the relationship areas and in three of the personal growth areas (all but the
open expression of anger) and relatively clear and well organized.
Again, staff control is low. The primary focus is on support, expressiveness, and clear and explicit policies. In general, these two sets of
programs seem to be well implemented, except perhaps for the lack of
structure in the TC programs.

Action-Oriented and Insight-Oriented Programs

Figure 4.3 presents the profile for the action-oriented programs,
which are high on autonomy and moderately high on staff control. All

FIGURE 4.3
WAS Form R Profiles for Patients in Action-Oriented and
Insight-Oriented Programs

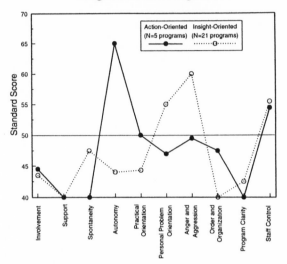

FIGURE 4.4
WAS Form R Profiles for Patients in Control-Oriented
and Undifferentiated Programs

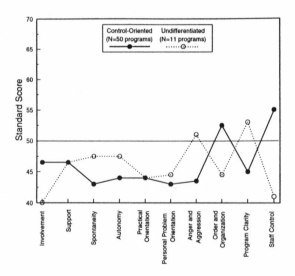

other WAS dimensions are average or below average. This cluster is composed of five high-turnover pre-release programs in which patients are expected to be independent and to make specific plans for their return to the community. However, the individualized program and high turnover rate are associated with a lack of involvement and cohesion and considerable confusion about program policies.

Figure 4.3 also shows the profile for the twenty-one programs in the insight-oriented cluster, which emphasizes self-understanding and the open expression of anger, but does so in a context that lacks involvement and support. Staff control is elevated; however, these programs lack organization and clarity. These insight-oriented programs have not established the type of supportive and self-directed climate in which patients can effectively enhance their self-understanding.

Control-Oriented and Undifferentiated Programs

A surprising total of fifty of the 144 programs fell into a control-oriented or custodial cluster. These programs emphasize organization and control. As shown in figure 4.4, they are below average in all other areas.

Eleven programs were placed in an undifferentiated cluster, which is also profiled in figure 4.4. Only anger and aggression and program clarity are above average. Most of these are state hospital admission programs with acutely disturbed or impulsive patients.

Size and staffing indices differentiated among these six types. The control-oriented programs were almost twice as large and only half as well staffed as the four treatment-oriented clusters. On average the control-oriented programs had about fifty-five patients and one staff member for each 7.6 patients, whereas the treatment-oriented clusters had about thirty patients and one staff member for each four patients. The undifferentiated programs were slightly larger than the TC programs but were almost as well staffed. Overall, the findings imply that a substantial proportion of programs are not well implemented with respect to the quality of patient-staff relationships or a balanced emphasis on performance expectations for patients and patients' personal growth.

An Intentional Social Systems Model of Care

As we have noted, projects designed to evaluate the differential outcome of treatment programs should include measures of the social environment; that is, of specific aspects of the actual treatment process that may influence patients to change. Such measures can help to specify the salient characteristics of a program, to compare two or more programs, and to ensure that the programs are implemented as planned. In this vein, we monitored an innovative attempt to design an intentional social systems program and compared it with a more traditional program (Moos, 1974; chapter 5).

The programs were on two adjacent physically identical thirty-bed units in a VA medical center. Patients were randomly assigned to the experimental or control unit and thus patients in the two programs were closely comparable. The patients were middle-aged (mean age about forty) and relatively well educated (average about twelve years). They had at least average work skills and income levels, although most had unstable employment histories and were alienated from former family relationships. On average, these patients had been hospitalized four times before; about half the patients had a current diagnosis of psychosis.

The basic goal of the experimental program was to design an intentional social systems treatment model by developing problem-solving task groups that involved a division of labor and interdependence among patients and staff. The program philosophy incorporated group membership, social processes, and tasks as core treatment elements; that is, the social system and task groups were seen as curative agents, not just as supportive of more specific treatment. The reorganization and development of patient-staff task groups involved the formation of a nonprofit corporation (Dann Services) for the delivery of psychiatric services; patients participated at all levels, including corporate directorships, management, and treatment.

The task groups included a patient-staff team that made decisions about patients' treatment plans and discharges, an employment workshop, and a community housing planning group. Patients who received services were also involved in delivering them. Although staff roles became more indirect and consultative, traditional treatment activities were also utilized. These included individual therapy, group therapy in the form of task groups, community meetings, recreational activities, and medication.

The primary innovation was in the emphasis on structured program elements provided by the task group orientation. The social system distributed decisionmaking power equally between patients and staff and furnished opportunities for patients to move into positions of responsibility and leadership. The program emphasized practical problem solving and crisis resolution. Theoretically, the program was based on the assumption that a change in patients' social behavior would lead to personality change and subsequently to better self-understanding.

The purpose of intentional social systems therapy is to create a treatment system that facilitates ego growth and mutually satisfying social behavior. The model is based on a synthesis of principles drawn from ego psychology, role theory, and organizational theory. By emphasizing a specific self-help orientation toward treatment, a program can become a supportive, problem-solving, self-maintaining social system, that is, an intentional community. In addition to transmitting enthusiasm and positive expectations for performance, the essential elements of the intentional social system are as follows:

- Meaningful, clearly specified tasks and roles are established, requiring interdependence and a division of labor among members. The tasks represent various degrees of complexity, challenge, and responsibility. Patients' roles approximate those required for normal living; their fulfillment is essential for the functioning of the system.
- The organizational structure provides for supportive group membership, participation in decisionmaking by all group members, graded responsibility, accountability, and a series of challenges for patients ranging from problems of everyday living to naturally occurring crisis situations.
- Incentives and group rewards are linked to task performance. Feedback on performance is provided for all members—staff and patients alike.
- Self-government by members is in accord with general standards of the community at large. Members' power to make policies and decisions regulating their own behavior requires living with the consequences of these decisions.
- To develop self-awareness, a sense of reality, and better interpersonal relationships, participants continually examine their interpersonal behavior and its consequences.

In contrast, the comparison program used a traditional model of treatment. Staff conceptualized the milieu or social system as supportive to more specific therapies. Formally these included medications, individual therapy, community meetings, recreational activities, and occupational therapy. The comparison program, which emphasized interpersonal relationships as the core of treatment, valued the staff team, the philosophy of participation and sharing, nursing care, and individual therapy. The "people equal program" slant meant that the program relied heavily on individual staff members' effectiveness, rather than on structural elements of the social system.

In this program, staff had decisionmaking power and delivered all treatment services directly. The focus was on individual patients and their personal goals were considered paramount. The underlying idea was that self-understanding and conflict resolution would promote personality change and subsequent change in social behavior. Employment placement generally followed the restoration of personality function and subsequent discharge from the program.

Development of the Intentional Social Systems Program

In the development phase, the social systems program had a coherent treatment environment; that is, the emphasis on the relationship and personal growth dimensions was average or above average. Compared with the comparison program, patients in the social systems program reported more practical orientation and open expression of anger, reflecting this program's emphasis on employment, outside community issues, confrontation, and the sharing of angry feelings. Comparison program patients noted more spontaneity, reflecting a more traditional concern with the expression of feelings per se, although not specifically angry feelings. Staff in the social systems program reported more emphasis on the personal growth dimensions, whereas comparison program staff reported more focus on the system maintenance dimensions.

Implementation and Stability of the Program

Figure 4.5 shows the treatment environment as seen by patients in the active phase of the project, by which time the social systems program was fully developed. Social systems patients reported more involvement and spontaneity than comparison patients did. They also reported more emphasis on autonomy, the development of social and work skills, and, to a lesser extent, self-understanding and the open

FIGURE 4.5
**WAS Form R Profiles for Patients in Social Systems
and Comparison Programs**

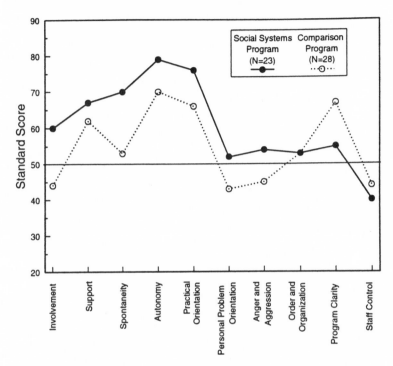

expression of anger. Staff in the social systems program also reported more emphasis on all four personal growth dimensions. However, social systems patients saw their program as somewhat less clear than comparison patients saw their program. In general, these program differences held for staff (not shown).

The social systems program was much more stable during the prior 8-month interval than the comparison program was. Patients and/or staff in the comparison program reported declines in involvement, practical orientation, and personal problem orientation, as well as in organization and staff control.

The changes in the comparison program corresponded to a period of leadership crisis, low staff morale, and low patient discharge rates. Only the emphasis on program clarity remained higher in the comparison program, probably reflecting its somewhat simpler and more familiar organization. A senior professional was planning on leaving the program, thus exposing its major weakness—the almost exclusive emphasis on "people as therapy" and the relative lack of concern with structured program elements such as the employment service group task.

The final profile for the social systems program revealed the remarkable stability of a well-implemented, structured program. The stability of this program from the initial to the final assessment, an interval of more than three years, is indicated by WAS profile correlations of .73 for patients and .96 for staff. This stability was achieved even though there was complete turnover of patients and substantial turnover of staff. In contrast, comparison program patients and staff reported less involvement, spontaneity, and practical orientation in the follow-up phase, indicating a further deterioration in this program.

Staff opinions about their program were solicited several times during the project. Social systems staff reported more positive reactions than comparison staff did. During the active evaluation phase, there were pronounced differences of opinion about patients' morale and enthusiasm and staff members' estimates of program effectiveness. Comparison program staff finally switched to the belief that the social systems program would have better results than their own program. In fact, the proportion of patients who worked full-time or part-time was about four times higher in the social systems than in the comparison program. The combination of slow patient turnover, a gradually accumulating group of chronic patients, and a comparatively small proportion of patients who worked or had job training resulted in the comparison program's staff members' more pessimistic views.

Assessment as Self-Analysis and Quality Control

This program comparison illustrates some applications of the assessment of treatment environments: examining program implementation, comparing programs, and monitoring program stability over time. The WAS provided a systematic description of the treatment environment, a description that closely corresponded to the different emphases in the programs. By comparing patient and staff groups with each other and over time, similarities and differences between programs and groups were identified.

The stronger focus on personal growth in the social systems program and on system maintenance in the comparison program, especially in the early phase of the project, reflected the social system program's emphasis on task groups, self-direction, the development of job skills, and self-understanding, as well as the comparison program's emphasis on the maintenance of a traditional treatment system. During this time, both programs had generally positive treatment environments and approximately equal discharge rates. Later changes in the comparison program were accompanied by a decline in discharge rates and in staff members' enthusiasm about their program's effectiveness.

There was a high degree of congruence between the WAS findings and other findings about the two programs, such as staff opinions about their programs, staff rankings of the importance of different treatment components, and analyses of the communications in the community meetings. For example, the social system program's community meetings emphasized problem solving and task orientation; they were highly structured, patient dominated, and decision oriented. The comparison program's community meetings were staff dominated and oriented toward discussing group and personal problems.

Patients discharged from the social systems program showed better work adjustment. A twelve- to eighteen-month follow-up showed 44 percent less accumulated rehospitalization among patients discharged from the social systems program and better work outcome: 270 versus 136 days worked on the first full-time job. However, patients in the comparison program had somewhat better symptom improvement: 51 percent of the social systems patients and only 36 percent of the comparison patients experienced high anxiety at twelve- to eighteen-month follow-up. In this regard, although the social systems program emphasized support and work skills, it also was oriented toward confrontation and the open expression of anger. Even though a generally satisfying environment was maintained and patients felt that the program enhanced their self-confidence, the program was relatively demanding and anxiety provoking.

This example shows that regular assessment of a treatment program can serve a valuable monitoring or quality control function. Congruence between patient and staff groups and/or between the actual and preferred environment is an important factor in effective program operation. Repeated measures of social system process over time provide the opportunity for self-analysis at both individual program and facility levels. Regular feedback of process data helps monitor the evolution and function of a system over time; in addition, it can be used to spot crises and to promote desired changes in program goals.

We have highlighted the considerable variation in the treatment environments of psychiatric and substance abuse programs in the United States and in other countries. To better understand how programs with varying treatment orientations influence patients' in-program and community outcomes, evaluation researchers need to assess how well they are implemented. If implementation is found wanting, the findings can be used to monitor and improve programs prior to an outcome evaluation. In the next three chapters, we focus on these issues as they apply to community programs.

Part II

Community Programs

5

The Social Climate
of Community Programs

Two main trends have contributed to a substantial growth in community residential programs in the past thirty years. One trend involved the reaction against custodial hospital care and the progressive move toward deinstitutionalization in which a large number of hospitalized patients were discharged to the community. Many of these patients were not able to function independently and needed a supportive residential setting to provide a place to live, an opportunity to socialize, useful vocational and avocational activities, and medical and mental health services. Accordingly, mental health practitioners evolved a set of models for psychosocial rehabilitation for chronically mentally ill individuals and a range of residential settings for such individuals, including board-and-care homes, halfway houses, community lodges, foster family homes, and satellite housing (Lamb, 1994; Stein, 1989).

A second, quite separate trend involved the development of board-and-care facilities and halfway houses for individuals with alcohol-related disorders (Blacker and Kantor, 1960; Cahn, 1969). At first, these facilities provided only meals and shelter, but, over time, they added group counseling and vocational services and trained staff, and many developed a culture oriented toward self-awareness and the principles of Alcoholics Anonymous (AA). A parallel development that grew out of a reaction against AA principles led to highly structured therapeutic community models of care for individuals with drug-related disorders. These models included Synanon, which emphasized confrontation and community (Kanter, 1972), and somewhat more eclectic programs such as Daytop Village (Sugarman, 1974) and Phoenix House (DeLeon, 1973).

These two trends have recently received renewed impetus because of the current emphasis on reducing health care costs, an attendant sharp decline in the number of admissions and the length of acute inpatient care, and intensive pressure to identify less expensive forms of community care. Thus, there has been a substantial rise in the number and diversity of residential facilities in the community.

Describing Community Programs

Information about the early history, treatment orientation, and client characteristics in community programs is available in descriptions of residential programs for psychiatric and substance abuse patients in the United States (Cahn, 1969; Glasscote, Gudeman, and Elpers, 1971; Keller and Alper, 1970; Wechsler, 1960) and of halfway houses and day hospitals in the United Kingdom (Apte, 1968; Farndale, 1961), and in case studies of specific facilities such as Rutland Corner House (Landy, 1960) and Woodley House (Doninger, Rothwell, and Cohen, 1963). Although these early reports provide only limited information about the process of treatment in these facilities, program evaluators have consistently emphasized the importance of the social environment in community programs.

In an intensive study of forty halfway houses, Raush and Raush (1968) contrasted sociological model programs that provide a therapeutic environment and medical model programs that provide a supportive but neutral environment with the idea that active treatment takes place elsewhere. They concluded that these variations substantially influenced the clients in these homes. In this respect, both Lamb and Goertzel (1972) and Wilder and his colleagues (1968) note how a social climate that emphasizes self-direction and high performance expectations can enhance residents' social and vocational functioning.

These emerging treatment orientations helped to foster a broader psychosocial rehabilitation model of community care based in part on the principles of moral treatment, the importance of vocational training, skills development methods drawn from social learning theory, and a goal of providing an integrated set of services that includes residential care (Liberman, 1988). In this respect, Rutman (1987) described four more specific models of rehabilitation. One approach involves a surrogate family or clubhouse model, such as Fountain House, in which members develop a supportive, participatory setting that provides a place to work and socialize and structure for their daily lives (Beard, Propst, and Malamud, 1982).

A second approach is the high expectancy or educational model that is more structured and emphasizes self-development and training programs in which clients are expected to progress toward specific, contracted performance goals. Clients typically receive services in a time-limited residential program and then move into less supervised settings. A third approach is a consumer-guided model in which clients sponsor and operate their own programs. One of the first examples of this model was the Lodge Program, in which patients obtained specialized training while in the hospital and then were discharged as a group into a client-directed, communal residence in the community (Fairweather et al., 1969). Finally, there is an intensive case management model in which clients receive individualized services that may involve components of the other three models.

Given the prevalence of community care and several well-differentiated models of care, there is a need for conceptually based measures of community programs' treatment environments. In some relevant work, Apte (1968) assessed the level of permissiveness or restrictiveness in halfway houses and found that clients in permissive houses were more likely to be discharged to an independent placement in the community. Garety and Morris (1984) developed a Management Practices Questionnaire (MPQ) to tap client versus management orientation; they found a strong client orientation in a hostel for chronically mentally ill individuals. Moreover, when Allen, Gillespie, and Hall (1989) applied the MPQ, they noted a stronger client orientation in a hospital than in a community program.

Based on these ideas and the growing importance of community programs in the continuum of psychiatric and substance abuse care, we proceeded to develop a method to assess the treatment environment of community residential programs. We had four main goals:

- to describe the diversity of community treatment programs on the three underlying sets of dimensions described earlier, that is, relationship, personal growth, and system maintenance dimensions;
- to compare different types of community programs, such as halfway houses, board-and-care homes, day hospitals, and sheltered workshops, as well as community with hospital programs;

- to develop a way to provide meaningful feedback to clients and staff about their treatment program and to help them improve it; and
- to examine the determinants and outcomes of community programs and to compare the findings with those obtained in hospital programs.

The Community-Oriented Programs Environment Scale (COPES)

Rationale and Development

We adapted many of the items in the initial form of the Community Oriented Programs Environment Scale (COPES) from the WAS. In addition, to obtain information about the applicability of items and to reword them as needed, we held discussions with staff members and managers who were familiar with existing community programs. We developed new items from program descriptions and interviews with clients and staff in community programs.

Our formulation of three sets of social climate dimensions guided the choice and wording of specific items. Each item had to identify a program's emphasis on interpersonal relationships (such as involvement), on an area of personal growth (such as autonomy), or on system structure (such as organization). For example, an emphasis on involvement is inferred from such items as: "Members put a lot of energy into what they do around here," and "This is a lively program." An emphasis on autonomy is inferred from such items as "Members are expected to take leadership here," and "Members here are very strongly encouraged to be independent." An emphasis on organization is inferred from such items as: "Members here follow a regular schedule every day," and "Members' activities are carefully planned." (There is no single adequate or generally accepted term for program participants. We use the words "client," "resident," and "member" interchangeably, but we prefer "member" because it has the broadest applicability and the most positive connotation.)

We administered the initial 130-item version of the COPES to members and staff in twenty-one community programs, selected to obtain a broad range of program types. The programs included nine day-care centers, four residential centers, two rehabilitation centers, three community care homes, a resident workshop, and two residential centers for youth. Most of the programs were open to women and men, but one house accepted only women and three accepted only men. About half the houses were transitional residences for psychiatric and/or substance abuse patients who had been discharged from hospital; the other half were designed to serve as an alternative to hospitalization. Most of the members were able to function moderately well and were eligible for full-time employment; one of the programs was composed of men with a history of chronic mental illness and was affiliated with a sheltered workshop. There was a wide range of structure in the programs. The centers for youth and the home for men were fairly structured and kept close control over their members, but many of the other programs allowed members a considerable amount of autonomy.

A total of 373 members and 203 staff in the twenty-one programs completed the COPES. As with the WAS, respondents answer each COPES item true if it characterizes the program and false if it does not. More than 80 percent of the members and essentially all the staff were able to complete the scale. We initially sorted items by agreement among three independent judges into twelve subscales paralleling the twelve initial WAS subscales (Moos, 1972a).

Psychometric Criteria and Final Form

To select items for the final form of the COPES, we applied five psychometric criteria.

- No more than 80 percent of respondents should answer an item in one direction (either true or false). This criterion eliminates items characteristic only of unusual treatment settings. Overall, 95 percent of the items met this criterion for members or staff or both.
- Items should correlate more highly with their own subscale than with any other. All of the final 100 items met this criterion. More specifically, more than 90 percent of the items for members and more than 95 percent for staff correlated above .30 with their appropriate subscales.
- Each subscale should have a nearly equal number of items scored true and items scored false to control for acquiescence response set. Of the ten subscales, four have five items scored true and five scored false; six subscales have six items scored true and four scored false.
- The subscales should have low to moderate intercorrelations. In fact, the average subscale intercorrelations are around .25, indicating that the subscales measure relatively distinct characteristics of community treatment programs.
- Each subscale should discriminate significantly among community programs. All ten subscales meet this criterion.

We also selected items that did not correlate significantly with a halo response set scale, which assessed positive and negative halo in residents' and staff members' program perceptions. Two of the original twelve subscales were dropped in the process of subscale development. The original variety subscale had low item-subscale correlations and showed poor internal consistency. Most of the items in the original affiliation subscale correlated as highly with other subscales (particularly involvement) as they did with affiliation.

The application of these criteria resulted in the ten-subscale COPES Real Form (Form R). Table 5.1 lists the subscales and gives brief definitions of each. The conceptualization of the dimensions is comparable to that for the WAS. The involvement, support, and spontaneity subscales measure relationship dimensions. The next four subscales (autonomy, practical orientation, personal problem orientation, and anger and aggression) are the personal growth dimensions. The last three subscales (order and organization, program clarity, and staff control) assess system maintenance dimensions. The complete COPES scoring key is in Appendix B.

The Diversity of Community Programs

Community Programs in the United States

We tried to develop an initial normative sample that included a diversity of community programs and represented several different alternatives to hospitalization. We surveyed fifty-four programs; both clients and staff were assessed in thirty-two programs and only clients were assessed in the remaining twenty-two programs.

The thirty-two programs in which we assessed both clients and staff include two rehabilitation workshops, two partial hospitalization programs, eleven halfway houses, and seventeen day-care centers. The workshops emphasized physical and occupational rehabilitation and primarily served individuals with relatively chronic psychiatric problems. The two partial hospitalization programs were administered by state hospital staff and admitted patients for either day or night care.

The halfway houses include three homes for youth, five homes for both women and men, one home for women only, and two homes for men only. These homes varied in capacity from five to thirty clients. All were managed by professionally trained psychologists or psychiat-

TABLE 5.1
COPES Subscale and Dimensions Descriptions

Relationship Dimensions

1.	Involvement	how active and energetic members are in the program
2.	Support	how much members help and support each other; how supportive the staff is toward members
3.	Spontaneity	how much the program encourages the open expression of feelings by members and staff

Personal Growth Dimensions

4.	Autonomy	how self-sufficient and independent members are in making decisions and how much they are encouraged to take leadership in the program
5.	Practical Orientation	the extent to which members learn social and work skills and are prepared for discharge from the program
6.	Personal Problems Orientation	the extent to which members seek to understand their feelings and personal problems
7.	Anger and Aggression	how much members argue with other members and staff, become openly angry, and display other aggressive behavior

System Maintenance Dimensions

8.	Order and Organization	how important order and organization are in the program
9.	Program Clarity	the extent to which members know what to expect in their day-to-day routine and the explicitness of program rules and procedures
10.	Staff Control	the extent to which the staff use measures to keep members under necessary controls

ric social workers whose role was to advise the live-in staff and to counsel the clients. Specifically designed to prepare their residents to live independently in the community, these programs typically discharged clients after six months to a year.

The seventeen day-care programs include four VA centers with about thirty members each, four programs affiliated with general or psychiatric hospitals, two county programs, and seven privately run programs with about fifteen members each. These programs were relatively well staffed and focused on improving self-care skills, interpersonal and social skills, and work skills.

The twenty-two programs in which we assessed only clients include twenty community care homes, a client-administered self-help program, and an outpatient support group. As a rule, between four and seven residents lived in the community care homes. There was a live-in foster parent who handled cooking, supervised housekeeping, and helped plan occasional trips for the residents. These facilities were meant to provide a supportive, homelike setting for residents who had had long-term hospitalizations and were able to function only at a minimal level. A few of the residents attended day-care centers or local sheltered workshops, but most remained at home during the day. Social workers consulted with foster parents about clients' behavior problems and held monthly meetings to help manage administrative matters.

The client-administered self-help program was run by an elected council that dealt with all administrative and behavior problems. The council screened and chose prospective clients. All clients had to work, go to school, or attend a day treatment center. The program was designed to prepare clients to live independently after a six-month period. The outpatient support group was composed of six former patients who met twice a week to discuss their mutual problems. Thus the initial normative sample includes a broad range of programs; the COPES was completed by a total of 778 members and 357 staff. The subscale means and standard deviations for the sample are provided in the COPES manual (Moos, 1996a).

Figure 5.1 shows the mean scores for members in fifty-four programs and staff in thirty-two programs. (In chapter 7 we compare the thirty-two programs with professional staff and the twenty-two programs with only paraprofessional staff.) On average, members and staff report comparable emphasis on the three relationship dimensions. Similar to

FIGURE 5.1
COPES Form R Means for Members and Staff
in Programs in the United States

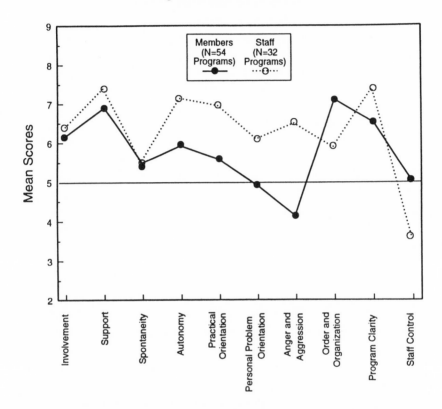

the patient-staff differences in hospital programs, staff in community programs report more emphasis on all four of the personal growth dimensions than members do. Compared with members, staff also appraise the programs as somewhat clearer and less controlling.

Overall, except on the relationship dimensions, staff see community programs somewhat more positively than clients do. The greater agreement on the relationship dimensions may reflect community programs' relatively small size and resultant communication between members and staff and the fact that clients in community programs are relatively healthy and participate with staff in program activities. Nevertheless, staff members' more positive perspectives about these programs is consistent with the greater responsibility staff members have for maintaining them.

In a project that involved the development of new procedures to assess facilities' physical features and policies and services, Timko (1995) obtained COPES data on sixty-two community programs. According to both members and staff, these programs, on average, were higher on involvement, support, and spontaneity than the programs in the original normative sample. In addition, they had a stronger focus on self-understanding and staff control. These differences probably reflect both a generational shift in treatment orientation toward more structure and the fact that Timko's (1995) sample includes a larger proportion of substance abuse programs.

Community Programs in the United Kingdom

We wanted the COPES to apply to community programs in countries other than the United States in order to be able to conduct cross-cultural comparisons of treatment programs. Accordingly, we applied the COPES to a sample in the United Kingdom (UK) composed of two day hospitals and eighteen halfway houses. The day hospitals, located at two major teaching hospitals in London, were characterized by high staff-client ratios and short-stay clients who were able to function in a limited manner in the community. One day hospital had fourteen clients and six staff; the other had twenty-one clients and twelve staff.

Three of the halfway houses were administered by the Borough of London. Each of these houses had between five and ten residents and each had three staff members. These programs were designed to help residents overcome substance abuse problems and usually allowed them to stay for six to twelve months.

The remaining fifteen halfway houses were administered by the Richmond Fellowship; these houses were oriented primarily toward residents' independence and vocational rehabilitation (Jansen, 1980). The houses ranged in size from four residents and one staff member to twenty-one residents and seven staff members. Residents in these programs were mostly young (mean age in the early twenties) and often were admitted by court referral. The programs encouraged residents to stay from six to twelve months. The Fellowship employs paraprofessional staff and has inservice training programs to maintain staff morale and help staff develop a consistent therapeutic orientation.

These programs are active and involving; they emphasize demo-

FIGURE 5.2
COPES Form R Means for Members and Staff in Programs
in the United Kingdom

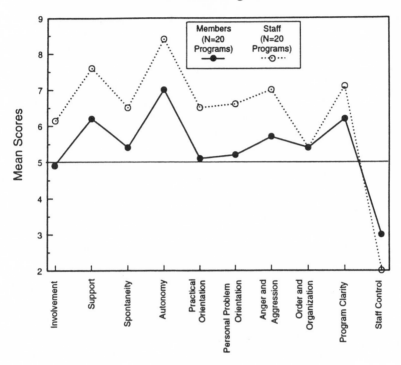

cratic decision-making processes. For example, residents vote on decisions that affect their life in the house; each resident and each staff
member receives one vote. The treatment program includes regular
weekly group sessions in which residents are encouraged to express
feelings about themselves and the staff. These sessions are well attended and tend to enhance resident-staff communication (Jansen, 1980).

A total of 209 residents and seventy-four staff members in the
twenty UK programs completed the COPES. Figure 5.2 shows the
COPES Form R profiles for these samples. The subscale means and
standard deviations are given in the COPES manual (Moos, 1996a).
As with the UK hospital sample, staff saw more emphasis on all three
relationship and all four personal growth dimensions than members
did. The group differences were somewhat less on the system mainte-

nance dimensions, although staff reported more focus on clarity and less on staff control than members did. The overall shape of the COPES profile is similar for members and staff. Moreover, both groups agree that these UK programs strongly emphasize members' self-reliance and independence—the highest score is on autonomy and the lowest is on staff control.

Although the programs in the United States and the UK differ somewhat in program characteristics and size, it is still instructive to compare them. Compared with their UK counterparts, residents in community programs in the United States see them as more involving and supportive, more oriented toward the development of work and social skills, and much more structured. Residents in UK programs report more emphasis on autonomy than residents in American programs do. These findings probably reflect differences in the samples of programs in the two countries, as well as a somewhat stronger emphasis on community care in the UK.

Psychometric and Methodologic Issues

Internal Consistencies and Intercorrelations

We calculated the internal consistencies of the ten COPES subscales, the average correlations between each item and its own subscale, and the average correlations between each item and the other nine subscales. All the subscales had acceptable internal consistency; Cronbach's alpha averaged .79 for residents and .78 for staff. In addition, the items correlated more highly with their own than with other subscales (Moos, 1974).

To discover whether it might be fruitful to work with a smaller number of dimensions, we intercorrelated the ten subscale scores separately for the 373 clients and the 203 staff in the American sample. The highest intercorrelation was .50; the only cluster of subscales that showed moderate intercorrelations in both the client and the staff samples was composed of the three relationship dimensions (Moos, 1974). The overall average correlation among the subscales was .23 for clients and .24 for staff. Thus the ten dimensions measure distinct but moderately related aspects of residents' and staff members' perceptions of community programs. In general, the subscale internal inconsistencies and intercorrelations are comparable for the larger normative samples that are currently available (Moos, 1996a).

Reliability, Profile Stability, and Differences among Programs

The COPES has adequate test-retest reliability and high profile stability. Profile stabilities were obtained by calculating rank-order correlations on the subscale standard scores for different administrations of the COPES in a set of diverse programs. In twenty-two readministrations of the COPES to clients over four- to nine-month intervals, the average profile stability was .82; in fifteen readministrations to staff the average stability was .80 (Moos, 1996a).

The profile stability of programs with a consistent treatment philosophy is very high over one- to two-year intervals; the average stability was .86 for thirteen readministrations to clients and .68 for sixteen readministrations to staff. These average profile stabilities are remarkable, because few if any of the same clients remained in these programs for intervals of six months or longer. Thus, the COPES measures aspects of the treatment climate that may remain stable despite a complete turnover in the client population. However, the COPES is also a sensitive measure of program change (chapter 6).

The results of one-way analyses of variance indicated that all ten subscales significantly differentiated among the twenty-one programs for both clients' and staff members' responses. According to Estimated Omega Squared, program differences accounted for an average of 20 percent of the subscale variance for clients' perceptions and 27 percent for staff members'. Thus, variations among programs account for a substantial proportion of the subscale variance.

Personal Characteristics and Program Perceptions

Researchers report few if any consistent relationships between personal factors and clients' perceptions of community programs. We found that clients' appraisals of substance abuse programs' treatment environments were essentially independent of demographic, psychosocial, personality, and alcohol-related functioning variables. Clients who were more highly educated had a tendency to evaluate their programs somewhat more negatively, whereas clients with fewer symptoms and less severe drinking problems tended to evaluate them somewhat more positively (Moos and Bromet, 1978; see also Cronkite and Moos, 1978). Pino and Howard (1984) found no association between the extent to which residents answered questions about themselves in a socially desirable direction and their program perceptions.

In a study of twenty-seven residential and thirty outpatient drug treatment programs, Friedman et al. (1986a) noted that women clients tended to rate their program more positively than men clients did; however, women staff rated it more negatively than did men staff. These differences may have been associated with clients' or staff members' minority status in these programs. Alternatively, because clients and staff were sampled from different programs, the findings may be due to program differences in treatment environments rather than to variations among individuals in the same program.

Staff Role and Perceptions of the Treatment Environment

Staff members, who have more responsibility for treatment programs, tend to see them more positively than clients do. Accordingly, we thought that specific groups of staff members who have more authority over program policies and treatment orientations, such as physicians and psychologists, might appraise them more optimistically than nurses or nurses aides. To examine this idea, we obtained some data on the role position of staff members who completed the WAS and the COPES.

Staff Role in Hospital Programs

In a sample of twenty-one hospital programs, one or more psychiatrists, nurses, and aides completed the WAS. There were some differences in how these three groups saw their treatment program; the largest differences were between psychiatrists and aides. Psychiatrists saw their program as more involving and supportive than either nurses or aides did; they also reported more emphasis on all four personal growth dimensions. In contrast, the aides reported the most emphasis on organization, clarity, and staff control (Moos, 1974; chapter 12).

We also compared four more groups of staff from another set of hospital programs: psychologists, social workers, psychiatric residents, and nursing students. Psychologists reported more emphasis on involvement and support and on all four personal growth dimensions; they also reported less staff control than did the other staff in their programs. Psychologists in these programs fulfilled key roles and had substantial responsibilities; thus, the findings support the idea that staff members who have more responsibility for a program tend to perceive it more positively.

Staff role differences were conceptually comparable but much larger in programs in the UK. Specifically, we compared residents or registrars, nurses, and aides in fourteen programs. In the UK, the registrars are physicians; they have the most responsible positions and make most of the important decisions about patients and day-to-day program policies. Consistent with their responsible roles, registrars saw their programs much more positively than did the nurses on all three relationship and all four personal growth dimensions; in turn, the nurses saw the programs more positively than the aides did.

Staff Role in Community Programs

We obtained comparable findings in community programs; that is, senior staff (administrators, psychiatrists, program directors) tended to see their treatment programs more positively than did nurses, aides, clerical helpers, and other affiliated staff (Moos, 1974; chapter 12). Taken together, the results suggest that staff who have more administrative responsibility for a program appraise it more positively than other staff do. We obtained similar findings in other settings. Specifically, staff see correctional facility social environments more positively than residents do (Moos, 1987), supervisors see work group climates more positively than do the employees they supervise (Moos, 1994c), and parents appraise family environments more optimistically than their adolescent children do (Moos and Moos, 1994a).

These findings have two important implications: (1) staff members are likely to benefit from an outside evaluation that enables them to share their views of their treatment program; and (2) brochures and other program descriptions should not be compiled solely by program administrators and directors. These individuals may present an overly optimistic picture of the treatment milieu, engendering unrealistically positive expectations among prospective clients. In turn, unrealistic expectations may foster some clients' disappointment and negative reactions to the program, poor adaptation to the program, and high dropout rates (see chapter 9).

Preferences about Community Programs

We reworded the COPES items to enable clients and staff to answer them in terms of their program preferences. The rationale for developing this Ideal Form (Form I) was comparable to the rationale for constructing the Ideal Form of the WAS. In fact, we could find no previously available techniques that assessed clients' and staff members' preferences about community programs' treatment environments. Again, Form I may be used with Form R to identify specific areas in which clients or staff think that change should occur (for more details, see chapter 6).

The COPES Form I is parallel to Form R; that is, each of the 100 items in Form I is parallel to an item in Form R. When completing Form I, clients and staff are asked to answer each item to describe an ideal program. We calculated item-subscale correlations and internal consistencies for the ten Form I subscales for a sample of fifteen programs. The average item-subscale correlations varied from .35 to .55; the subscale internal consistencies, which varied from .70 for clarity to .88 for personal problem orientation, are quite acceptable for both the client and staff samples. The Form I instructions and items are provided in the COPES manual (Moos, 1996a).

Preferences in the United States

Most of the American programs assessed with the COPES Form R were also assessed with Form I. Specifically, Form I was completed by clients in forty-seven of the fifty-four programs and by staff in twenty-six of the thirty-two programs assessed with Form R. A total of 618 clients and 252 staff completed Form I. The Form I norms are given in the manual (Moos, 1996a).

According to figure 5.3, clients and staff members in American community programs have relatively similar preferences, although staff see an ideal program as higher on all three relationship and all four personal growth dimensions. The differences between clients and staff in the community programs are quite similar to those between patients and staff in hospital programs (see figure 2.4). Compared to clients, staff want treatment programs to be more involving and supportive and to have higher performance expectations for clients.

Some important findings emerge when the results for the COPES Real Form (figure 5.1) are compared with those for the COPES Ideal Form (figure 5.3). On average, clients and staff want more emphasis on all three relationship dimensions and on autonomy, skills development, and self-understanding than currently exists in their program. They also prefer more order and clarity. In contrast, they are basically

FIGURE 5.3
COPES Form I Means for Members and Staff
in Programs in the United States

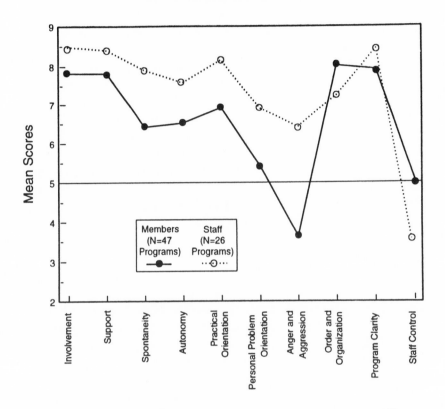

satisfied with the emphasis on the expression of anger and staff control.

Preferences in the United Kingdom

The COPES Form I was given to clients and staff in nineteen of the twenty programs in the UK; 176 clients and fifty-five staff completed the scale. As shown in figure 5.4, clients and staff in the UK conceptualize ideal treatment programs quite similarly. Staff want somewhat more emphasis on the relationship and personal growth dimensions, but the differences are somewhat smaller than those we identified in the American sample.

A comparison of figures 5.2 and 5.4 indicates that clients in UK

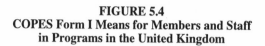

FIGURE 5.4
COPES Form I Means for Members and Staff
in Programs in the United Kingdom

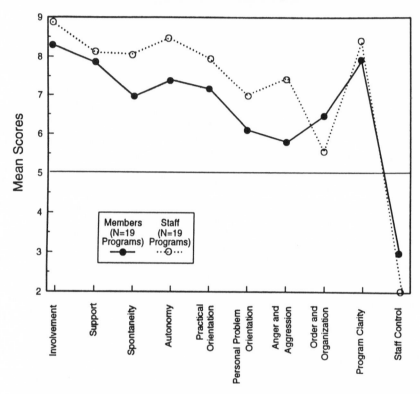

programs want much more emphasis than they have in most areas, particularly on the relationship dimensions and on practical orientation, organization, and clarity. Similarly, staff want more focus on involvement, spontaneity, and practical orientation.

We have described the rationale and development of the COPES, which assesses the treatment environment of community programs on ten dimensions that are conceptually comparable to those we use to assess hospital programs. The findings show that the COPES has adequate psychometric properties and that it can be applied to community programs in the United States and the United Kingdom. We turn next to the use of the scale in monitoring and improving programs.

6

Monitoring and Improving
Community Programs

We designed the COPES as a multipurpose evaluation procedure to characterize community treatment programs, focus on differences between residents' and staff members' perceptions of programs, and monitor stability and change in a program over time. We also wanted to use the COPES to provide feedback to staff and to help improve programs. These ideas are closely comparable to the applications of the WAS in hospital programs (chapters 3 and 4). To illustrate these applications, we provide examples of COPES profile interpretations and describe staff members' reactions to COPES feedback. We then focus on the accuracy of program descriptions and the use of the COPES to monitor program change and promote program improvement.

Interpreting Profiles and Providing Feedback

As with the WAS, the COPES can provide important information about a community program's treatment environment. To illustrate, we compare the COPES profiles for members and staff in Harbor Lights, a residential center for adults, and in Shady Glen, a community care home, to the American normative sample of fifty-four programs. In the same way as for the WAS, scores for members and staff are plotted in relation to members' norms.

FIGURE 6.1
COPES Form R Profiles for Members and Staff in Harbor Lights

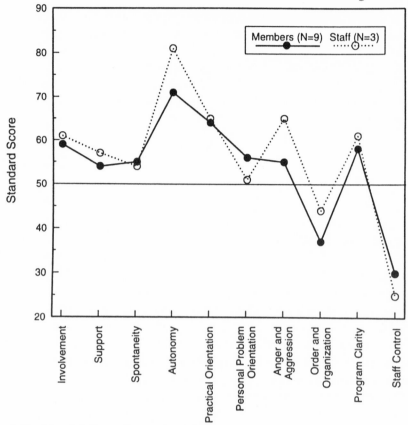

A Residential Care Center for Adults

Harbor Lights is a small, coeducational residential center for adults who are in crisis situations or are returning to the community after hospitalization. Clients are involved in regular daytime activities and are responsible for housework and cooking. They attend house management and group therapy meetings and are encouraged to be as independent as possible. Rules and restrictions are minimized. The house is staffed by a resident manager, a part-time student manager, and a program director. The staff consult with visiting social workers.

Figure 6.1 shows the COPES profiles for members and staff. Both groups reported somewhat above average emphasis on the relationship dimensions. For example, members and staff reported that discussions in the house were involving and that residents often planned weekend activities together.

Members and staff also agreed on the type of treatment orientation and structure in the program. Both groups reported a strong emphasis on independence and on learning social and work skills. Self-understanding and the expression of anger were given a lower priority. Members and staff saw the rules as clear and explicit but felt that the program was poorly organized and that staff did not adequately control it.

A Community Care Home

Shady Glen is a small community care home for women who have been discharged from hospital treatment and are trying to resume community living. It is located in a comfortable home in an urban residential area. The women may go to work, school, or a day-care center. The house is managed by two women who act as house mothers and encourage the residents to participate in community activities; two additional staff serve as administrative consultants.

As shown in figure 6.2, Shady Glen exemplifies a different type of treatment environment. There is a moderate level of disagreement between members and staff, especially on the relationship dimensions. Members rated involvement and spontaneity as about average, whereas staff rated them as well below average. For example, all four members felt that they participated actively in the program, but all four staff disagreed. Members rated support as very high, but staff saw it as only slightly above average.

Members and staff agreed more closely on the program's main treatment goals. Both groups reported a strong emphasis on the development of social and work skills and noted that self-direction and self-understanding were played down. In addition, there was very little open expression of anger. Members and staff viewed the program as especially clear and well-organized and agreed that staff control was about average.

Taken together, these two profiles show how the COPES can identify the salient aspects of a community treatment program with respect to normative standards of program implementation. Harbor Lights emphasizes autonomy and has few formal activities or rules. Residents are highly involved and communicate openly with one another. In

FIGURE 6.2
COPES Form R Profiles for Members and Staff in Shady Glen

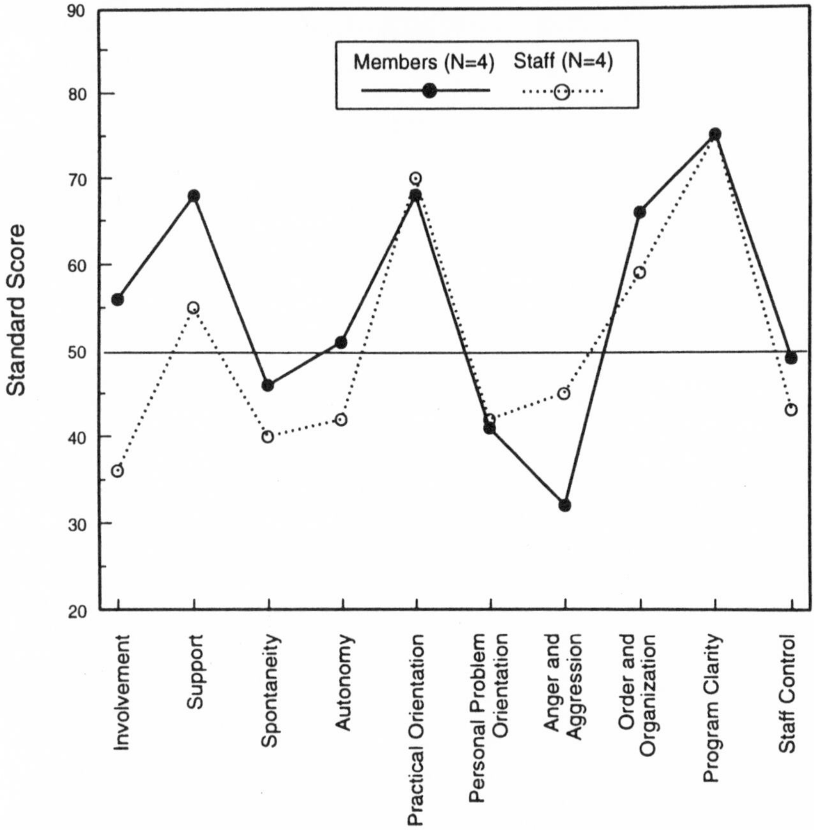

contrast, Shady Glen emphasizes support and practical orientation and provides a substantial level of structure.

Staff Reactions to COPES Feedback

We distributed feedback questionnaires in ten programs to evaluate the informational value and practical implications of the COPES profiles. The majority of staff reported that the COPES profiles portrayed their treatment program relatively accurately and completely. In addition, more than 80 percent reported that the COPES suggested important potential program changes.

The COPES enables staff to accurately describe their program on the basis of residents' as well as their own perceptions. Staff members often engage in an informed and critical analysis as they examine their own and the residents' preferences and compare them to the actual program. The COPES serves to guide the discussion. As a result of feedback, staff often identify specific changes that can improve their program. This application of the COPES as an analytic tool is comparable to the work done with the WAS (see chapter 3). In both cases staff learn that the evaluation process can be informative and can suggest specific practical solutions to problems in their program.

Evaluating Program Descriptions

The continuing growth of new types of psychiatric programs, especially community programs, has increased the need for more accurate and complete program descriptions. Because the treatment environment is an integral part of the therapeutic process, these descriptions should provide information about this aspect of the program. Knowledge about a program's social climate is important for prospective patients and staff, for referral and other community agencies, and for individuals interested in new developments in the field.

The program descriptions that have been written to fill these needs have depended primarily on program manager's appraisals, supplemented by surveys that cover physical features, staff and residents' characteristics, and treatment orientation. It is important to determine whether such published descriptions give an adequate picture of a program's treatment environment. To focus on this issue, we examined the published descriptions of a sample of community programs and used the COPES to evaluate the information presented about the treatment milieu (Otto and Moos, 1973).

We found published descriptions of five community programs for which COPES profiles for residents and staff were also available. We asked each of ten judges to complete the COPES for each program on the basis of the information in these descriptions. To measure how accurately the program's treatment milieu could be inferred from the published description, we compared the judges' perceptions with those of residents and staff in the program.

Judgments of the Five Programs

Program 1 is a coed center for residents who manage their daily affairs, take their own medications, and assist with housework. Three meetings a week are held to discuss residents' problems, assign work, and develop social skills. Program 2 is a residential center for men who attend a day hospital or receive training in vocational rehabilitation. The house provides a weekly group therapy session and some recreational activities. Program 3 is a residential center for youth who are referred from the courts or local state hospital. The youth attend public school; the program provides group and individual therapy. Program 4 houses chronically ill men who learn basic skills such as personal care and housekeeping and are given jobs in a specially supervised workshop. These four programs are described in *Halfway Houses for the Mentally Ill* (Glasscote, Gudeman, and Elpers, 1971).

The fifth program is a day treatment center. Members are expected to participate in confrontive group therapy and to enhance their social skills and independence by developing a therapeutic community. This program is described in *Partial Hospitalization for the Mentally Ill* (Glasscote et al., 1969).

According to the judges, there were significant differences among the five programs on nine of the COPES subscales (all except clarity). Thus, the written descriptions clearly gave different impressions of the programs' treatment milieus. We calculated intraclass profile correlations between the judges' COPES profiles and the residents' and staff members' profiles.

The judges' perceptions matched those of the residents and staff in programs 2 and 5 relatively well. The intraclass correlations were .70 and .71 for program 2 and .51 and .74 for program 5. However, the level of agreement was much lower for the coed residence, the residential center for youth, and the home for chronically ill men. For these three programs, the intraclass correlations averaged .25 for judges and residents and .22 for judges and staff. Thus, two of the reports provided more accurate information about the treatment environment than the other three did.

Accurate and Inaccurate Descriptions

There was good agreement between judges and program participants about program 5. The article was written on the basis of interviews with the program managers and staff; accordingly, the judges agreed with staff members' perceptions somewhat more than with residents' perceptions.

The published description explains that each resident is assigned to a committee that is responsible for making home visits, doing housework, maintaining and furnishing the home used for the center, and organizing social activities. There are daily community meetings and twice a week each resident participates in smaller, patient-led group therapy meetings. In addition, there are special interest groups for youth, women, and individuals with specific hobbies. The article explains that there is only one hour of free time a day. This description depicts a very active center with involved members. In fact, judges agreed with residents and staff on all ten of the involvement scale items.

Autonomy was another area in which judges agreed closely with participants. The committees mentioned earlier reflect the responsibilities residents are expected to assume; in addition, several sections in the published description focus on the high level of patient autonomy in the program.

The judges' scores strongly resembled those of the residents and staff in one of the men's residence programs (program 2), as well. In the area of practical orientation, the article explained that the program takes a life-management approach, emphasizing learning to handle everyday problems rather than focusing on gaining insight into personal problems. In the area of organization, the article mentioned that the house is kept clean and that residents are taught to be well groomed; it also listed organized daytime activities. Accordingly, judges agreed with residents and staff on the majority of the items on the practical orientation and organization subscales. Because the published description explained that the program's goal was to prepare the men for independent living, the judges agreed with residents and staff on four items relating to autonomy.

In contrast, the judges showed little or no agreement with residents or staff in their perceptions of the residential program for youth (program 3). The description noted the provision of group therapy and feedback sessions, but did not cover what was discussed or how these sessions contributed to residents' support. The description also explained that better functioning residents are moved to an adjacent house and have more privileges, but the specific privileges were not identified. Primarily the article discussed residents' demographic characteristics, eligibility, and common problems with drugs and family.

Judges agreed with residents and staff on more items for articles that supplied detailed discussions of the program philosophy and treatment orientation, and specific information about resident-staff interaction patterns. The length of the description was not the determining factor. However, one program for which judges and staff showed high agreement included several quotations from the program director and presented accounts of specific incidents at the center.

Guidelines for Writing Program Descriptions

Descriptions of treatment programs should provide as accurate and complete a picture as possible of these programs' essential characteristics. One major reason for inaccurate program descriptions is that important information about the program is left out. In addition, the description may present the program in an overly optimistic light because it is written by an individual who is responsible for the program and wants it to be seen in a positive way.

Program descriptions should include basic information about the institutional context and structure of a program, such as its size, staffing, cost, and so on. In addition, it is useful to provide information about the treatment climate and about each of the main sets of determinants of the climate; that is physical features, policies and services, and the aggregate characteristics of residents and staff.

Each of these four sets of dimensions provides a somewhat different perspective on a program; the use of all four should furnish relatively accurate and complete program descriptions. Because members and staff may have divergent views of a program, program descriptions should include both perspectives. Accounts of illustrative incidents in a program often add specificity to these aspects of program descriptions.

Inclusion of the type of information we have suggested can lead to the development of more complete and accurate program descriptions, which should be useful to counselors who need to make referral decisions, to prospective staff considering working in a particular program, and to program managers and evaluators who need to know about the range of existing programs in a community. Finally, clients themselves would gain, especially the growing proportion of clients who wish to take a more active part in choosing the treatment program that might be most beneficial for them.

Monitoring Program Change

As we described with respect to hospital programs (chapter 3), information about the treatment environment can be used to monitor the process of change in community programs. The COPES has been applied to examine a wide variety of changes, such as enhancing personal growth and structure in a halfway house, the development of new treatment orientations such as a teaching family program, and the reorientation of a psychodynamic program oriented toward self-understanding to a social rehabilitation program focused primarily on the development of work skills.

Enhancing Personal Growth and Structure in a Halfway House

We monitored the process of maturation and change in Pathways, a halfway house for individuals with substance abuse problems. When the COPES was first administered, Pathways was a newly established, sixteen-bed, long-term recovery home. Residents and staff had very similar perceptions of it, as shown in figure 6.3. Both groups saw strong emphasis on the relationship dimensions, especially involvement and spontaneity, and above average emphasis on independence, concern about personal problems, and the open expression of anger. Staff reported somewhat above average emphasis on practical orientation, but patients disagreed. However, residents and staff agreed that organization, clarity, and staff control were below average. Both groups portrayed a program that was relatively well implemented in the relationship and personal growth domains but somewhat lacking in system maintenance compared to normative conditions in other programs (Bliss, Moos, and Bromet, 1976; Moos et al., 1990).

A more individualized method for generating an implementation standard is to identify an ideal form of the intervention. As described earlier, Form I of the COPES allows residents and staff to specify their preferences about the treatment milieu. Figure 6.4 illustrates the changes residents and staff wanted in the Pathways program. The amount of change desired is obtained by subtracting the average score for the actual program from the average score for an ideal program for each subscale. The line marked zero in the center of the profile indicates no change is desired, or no discrepancy between the actual and preferred program. Positive scores indicate a desire for more emphasis, whereas negative scores point to a wish for less.

FIGURE 6.3
COPES Form R Profiles for Members and Staff in Pathways
—First Assessment

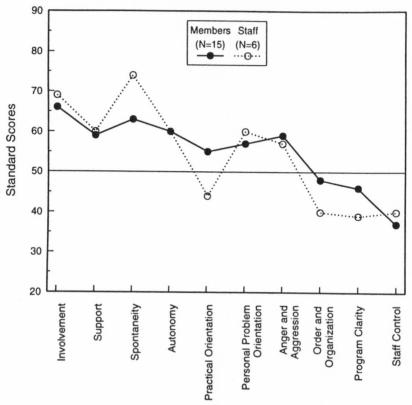

Residents and staff in Pathways saw a need for more emphasis on all aspects of the program. Staff wanted more spontaneity than residents did, whereas residents preferred more open expression of anger. Overall, staff preferred a clear and orderly program characterized by supportive relationships and an emphasis on the development of daily living skills and self-understanding. They did not wish to be faced with the management problems that might ensue from placing priority on resident autonomy and the open display of anger. Thus, aspects of a program that are judged to be well implemented on the basis or normative data, such as involvement and spontaneity, may be found wanting when compared to residents' and staff members' preferences.

Several developments took place in the subsequent six months. The original sixteen-person community was expanded to twenty-seven, and

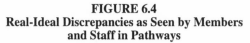

FIGURE 6.4
Real-Ideal Discrepancies as Seen by Members
and Staff in Pathways

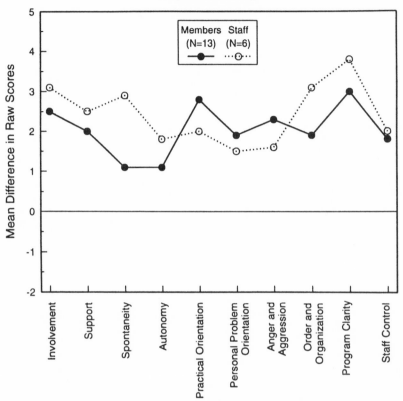

a more experienced director and new house manager were hired to stabilize the program. A new individualized recovery program allowed residents more freedom to plan activities suited to their needs. This led to an increase in the number of residents who accepted paid or volunteer work with community agencies or found regular part- or full-time employment. Transactional analysis became a major treatment modality and the number of therapeutic activities increased.

The interim treatment milieu. We readministered the COPES to residents and staff to identify the impact of these changes. Involvement and support diminished, reflecting the increase in program size and a corresponding decline in the quality of relationships among residents. House meetings were appraised as more businesslike, and the program became less intimate and more routine. The focus on practical orientation increased as more residents participated in vocational activities. Staff reported more emphasis on independence and self-understanding, as expected from the new priority on individualized recovery and transactional analysis. Clarity and staff control were augmented by the more defined program structure and the program director's and house manager's leadership. Thus, the changes in the treatment milieu followed predictably from the changes in the program.

More developments took place in the subsequent eight months. Staff gave the more experienced residents responsibility for leading group sessions and counseling new members. Changes in the admissions procedure enabled new residents to participate more actively. Community meetings were organized more clearly, and effective lines of communication were established to consider residents' ideas and grievances. In addition, the administrators became more actively involved in the day-to-day aspects of the program and added several new activities and therapy groups.

Longer-term program development. The COPES was readministered to residents and staff about eight months after the second assessment, or fifteen months after the initial assessment. The strengthened priority on vocational activities and employment led to a rise in practical orientation (figure 6.5). The insight-oriented treatment groups and the focus on transactional analysis stimulated a substantial increase in personal problem orientation. Residents and staff reported more organization and clarity as the new director stabilized the program structure and they became familiar with the new routine.

Pathways started out as an involved and supportive program. Nevertheless, involvement increased somewhat as residents participated more fully in the program by making decisions about how grievances should be resolved and by selecting new members. Staff members' perceptions of support were enhanced by the administrators' increased responsiveness, the senior residents' counseling role, and improved communication among residents, but these changes had not yet had an impact on residents' perceptions.

The changes in the halfway house program reflect a dynamic and involved pattern of maturation. Initially, the program was a small, close-knit community with moderate emphasis on treatment goals and relatively little structure. The overall program moved toward the residents' and staff members' preferred treatment milieu, that is, more

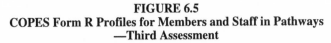

FIGURE 6.5
COPES Form R Profiles for Members and Staff in Pathways
—Third Assessment

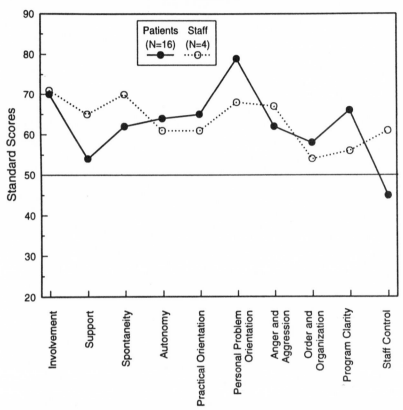

clarity and organization and somewhat more emphasis on the relationship and personal growth dimensions. However, some aspects of the
program still remained unsettled, as shown by the high level of anger
and the discrepancy between residents' and staff members' views of
clarity and staff control.

Development of a Teaching Family Program

In most group homes for youth, several part- and full-time staff
members work regular eight-hour shifts and share child management,
casework, and supervisory responsibilities. These staff members' roles
often overlap and their unique functions are not clearly defined. In

contrast, in the teaching family model, husband and wife couples (family teachers) live in the home on a 24-hour basis and provide a family milieu in which the youth are taught social, self-help, academic, and vocational skills. The family teachers also provide casework and counseling services. In this model of care, child and youth care workers fulfill a role of "therapeutic parents" that combines principles of psychotherapy and child and adolescent development (Shealy, 1995).

Schneider et al. (1982) examined the development of a teaching-family program in two group homes for youth. Both the youth and staff reported the social climate to be more closely aligned with ideal teaching-family principles after the program was changed. Specifically, both groups appraised the programs as more involving and supportive, more oriented toward personal growth, and clearer and better organized. Consistent with these changes, external evaluators reported an increase in program quality and the youth appraised staff as more pleasant and effective. Because staff had clearer and more stringent expectations for the youths' performance, the youth felt they were making more progress and their problem behavior declined; however, they were somewhat less happy in the new program.

Reorienting a Psychodynamic to a Rehabilitation Model

In a series of studies, Ryan and Bell (1983) monitored the process whereby staff changed a traditional psychodynamic program into a rehabilitation program with a strong emphasis on the development of vocational and work skills.

The Intensive Psychotherapy Program. The original program, a long-term, psychodynamically oriented Intensive Psychotherapy Program, emphasized self-understanding, the open expression of anger, and staff control. However, it was not supportive, clear, or well organized and it lacked an emphasis on self-direction and the development of work and social skills. Psychodynamic concepts guided the therapeutic community's activities and the staff's management and control of patients. This program was composed primarily of patients with schizophrenic disorders, and, as might be expected, these patients showed little overall improvement.

The investigators examined the changes that occurred during the four years when the Intensive Psychotherapy Program was modified first into the Therapeutic Residential Treatment Center (TRTC), a program that augmented psychodynamic treatment with self-help groups and social rehabilitation services in a therapeutic community framework. The TRTC was later replaced by the Veterans Resource Program (VRP), which was devoted primarily to the development of specific social, vocational, and community living skills.

The Veteran's Resource Program. As a psychosocial rehabilitation program that embodies a model for providing psychiatric rehabilitation services in a hospital setting, the Veterans Resource Program (VRP) entails a paid work program or part-time employment in industry. Patients learn specific skills in structured workshops and are encouraged to practice these skills in social clubs and community groups. To prepare for independent community living, patients work with a counselor to arrange appropriate housing and job placements. To help develop self-respect and autonomy, residents are referred to as veterans rather than patients. Moreover, there is a self-governing body called the Veterans Alliance; the veterans are entirely responsible for their own conduct in the evenings and nights and on weekends when no staff are on duty.

Thirteen administrations of the COPES at four-month intervals revealed substantial and predictable changes in the quality of the treatment environment, including increases in support, an orientation toward self-direction and skills development, and a decline in emphasis on self-understanding and staff control. These changes closely mirrored the conceptual differences between the psychodynamically oriented Intensive Psychotherapy Program and the rehabilitation-oriented Veterans' Resource Program model (Ryan, Bell, and Metcalf, 1982).

Bell and Ryan (1984) compared the Veterans' Resource Program with a high-quality, intensive acute inpatient program that referred patients to the VRP. The two programs were comparable on the relationship and system maintenance dimensions, even though the VRP staff worked only during the day. The VRP was seen as oriented much more strongly toward independence and skills training, whereas the referring unit was seen as more concerned with patients' personal problems and the maintenance of order.

Compared with baseline data and with residents treated in the Intensive Psychotherapy and TRTC programs, VRP residents had substantially lower dropout and six- and twelve-month relapse rates and were more likely to be employed at follow-up. These findings suggest that it may be more effective to develop a separate rehabilitation unit than to offer rehabilitation as an adjunct service on an intensive treatment unit or perhaps even than to refer inpatients directly to rehabilitation programs in the community.

Ideology and practice in rehabilitation programs. In a conceptual analysis of their findings, Bell and Ryan (1985) speculated that milieu treatment has a coherent ideology across programs and that ideology and practice are more compatible in programs focused on rehabilitation than in those with either a psychodynamic or a medical orientation. They formulated these conclusions from COPES profiles of the rehabilitation oriented and psychodynamically oriented programs and of a medically oriented program. Staff in the three programs saw the ideal treatment milieu similarly, though staff in the rehabilitation program preferred somewhat more autonomy and somewhat less personal problem orientation. Only in the rehabilitation milieu were there no significant discrepancies between the actual and preferred treatment environment: these findings imply that the treatment milieu was implemented adequately in the rehabilitation program but not in the other two programs.

Psychosocial rehabilitation units can be structured in line with the precepts of moral treatment. In this vein, Appelbaum and Munich (1986) described the transformation of two psychotherapy-based units for chronic schizophrenics and patients with severe character disorders into a rehabilitation program based in part on moral treatment ideals. The psychotherapy model emphasized understanding patients' psychodynamics, discussing staff members' feelings in team meetings, and employing an egalitarian decisionmaking process. To implement the rehabilitation model, decisionmaking power was redistributed such that patients and staff worked jointly to design treatment plans. While some staff responded negatively to the redefinition of roles, positive results included more supportive relationships among patients, greater patient autonomy, increased patient participation in therapeutic activities, and more emphasis on the restoration and development of patients' social and vocational skills.

Promoting Program Improvement

Program evaluators can use information obtained by the COPES to facilitate program development. Before trying to improve the social climate in a treatment program, it is important to understand the program, to outline the process of implementing change, and to anticipate potential problems. Program evaluators often collaborate with managers in these activities.

Steps in Assessing and Changing Treatment Programs

Here, we provide a brief outline of eight steps involved in the process of assessing and changing treatment programs:

1. *Develop an overview of the change program.* What are its objectives? How can the changes be accomplished? Who needs to be involved in the planning?
2. *Establish an assessment plan.* What elements in the program need to be evaluated? What is the anticipated time frame for the assessment? How will communications with the residents and staff be handled?
3. *Introduce the assessment to participants.* Give the reasons for the assessment. Outline the possible uses of the treatment climate information.
4. *Conduct the assessment.* Include relevant groups and administer the COPES. Possibly give individuals the option to respond anonymously. Possibly use interviews and other forms of data collection.
5. *Analyze and interpret the assessment results.* Compare different groups of residents and staff. Identify the nature and causes of any problems. Develop objectives and procedures for an intervention if necessary.
6. *Give feedback to participants.* Provide feedback in a form that residents and staff can understand. Consider giving residents and or staff opportunities to discuss the results.
7. *Plan and implement the change program.*
8. *Reassess the treatment environment.* Prior to reassessment, allow adequate time for changes to occur. Give feedback of new results to residents and/or staff. Fine-tune change programs as needed.

Improving a Residential Center for Youth

To show how feedback of COPES results can help to change a program, we conducted a study in Safehaven, a coeducational residential center for youth. The youngsters were diagnosed as having primarily mental or emotional difficulties; many also had substance abuse problems and a history of failure in school. The program had a capacity to serve fourteen youth; it had a director and four live-in staff members. Residents stayed in the program for about four months and progressed through four step levels; each level had more responsibilities and privileges. Residents were rated weekly on a point system by other residents and staff. Residents' progress was evaluated in such areas as personal care, money management, interpersonal relationships, and meeting performance expectations. There was a resident government, and the residents took responsibility for housekeeping and cooking (Moos, 1973; Moos, 1974, chapter 11).

Initial program perceptions. Figure 6.6 shows the initial COPES Form R profiles for the residents and staff. Both groups reported considerable emphasis on self-understanding and the open expression of anger. The residents also reported relatively strong focus on learning social and work skills; however, they saw the program as lacking in support and organization. Staff saw the program as strongly oriented toward independence, but residents disagreed.

According to the COPES Form I, both residents and staff wanted more emphasis on the quality of relationships, especially involvement and spontaneity, and on program organization and clarity. Both groups wanted less emphasis on the expression of anger.

Planning and promoting change. After a program evaluator discussed the profiles with residents and staff, both groups showed an interest in changing the treatment environment. The evaluator met with residents and staff over a four-month period to help them formulate specific modifications to the program. Three issues kept recurring.

Issues of autonomy and staff control were central, especially because residents saw much less self-direction in the program than staff did. The residents wanted more independence. Staff members' main concern was that residents typically asked them to make minor decisions that residents could make for themselves, such as whether or not they should go to school when they were sick. Staff also felt that residents had visions of having total freedom to do whatever they wanted without any concurrent responsibility.

Some staff felt that residents wanted support for their impulsive actions, but staff wanted to discourage such behavior. Accordingly, staff developed a specific procedure to enable residents to obtain support from their peers when they had a personal problem. Any resident could call a "game" whenever necessary. The other residents would then talk with the individual about the problem and help seek a solution that would not entail impulsive or disturbed behavior. For example, one girl called a "game" after she had an upsetting fight with her boyfriend.

There was a need to plan some enjoyable activities for the residents.

FIGURE 6.6
COPES Form R Profiles for Members and Staff in Safehaven
—Initial Assessment

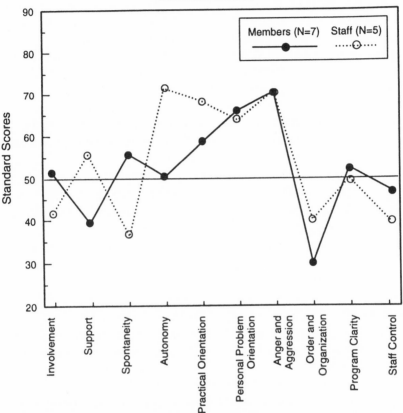

The program relied too heavily on problem-solving activities, which dampened residents' and staff members' enthusiasm.

To address these issues, the program evaluator and staff initiated several specific changes. To increase autonomy, one of the residents was named the work group supervisor and was given responsibility for organizing assigned tasks and checking to be sure that residents were completing their work adequately. Staff hoped that this change would clarify each resident's responsibilities and that staff would not need to continually check to ensure that tasks were actually completed.

A position of resident food manager was established. The food manager was responsible for checking menus and for making sure that the residents who were cooking dinner knew how to fix the meal and had all the supplies they needed.

The staff clarified the role of the resident coordinator and enlarged the sphere of responsibility of this position. The coordinator, who supervised both the work group supervisor and the food manager, was given the authority to call resident meetings whenever problems arose. In addition, he or she was placed on the screening committee, which made decisions about accepting new residents. As might be expected in a residential center for youth, autonomy and staff control issues were quite complex and were discussed in detail.

Residents and staff hoped that these changes would result in increased involvement, autonomy, and clarity. Several additional attempts were made to clarify staff members' expectations of residents—for example, giving a resident responsibility for teaching new residents their job obligations, developing a clearer structure in the process of individual goal setting, and establishing a new procedure by which each resident rated the other residents on certain personal characteristics. Staff also instituted a procedure whereby new residents met with the director to focus on specific problem areas and set measurable goals.

Changes in program perceptions. To track program changes, we gave COPES Forms R and I to residents and staff about six months after the initial assessment. Figure 6.7 summarizes the changes in real-ideal program discrepancies. Points above the zero line indicate that residents or staff saw the program as closer to their preferences at the second assessment, whereas points below the zero line indicate that the program was further away from their preferences.

The residents saw the treatment milieu as closer to their preferences at the second assessment. The program became more involving and supportive, oriented toward residents' self-direction, and clear and well organized. For example, residents were more likely to report that the program had sufficient social activities, that residents were given enough individual attention, that there was an active resident government, and that staff almost always acted on residents' suggestions. The staff also saw the program as closer to their preferences at the second assessment, especially in terms of involvement and clarity. Thus specific changes occurred in each of the four major areas that were discussed following the initial feedback sessions.

Importantly, residents' and staff members' preferences for personal problem orientation and the expression of anger declined. Because preferences may evolve during feedback and discussion sessions, a

FIGURE 6.7
COPES Form R Profiles for Members and Staff in Safehaven
—Third Assessment

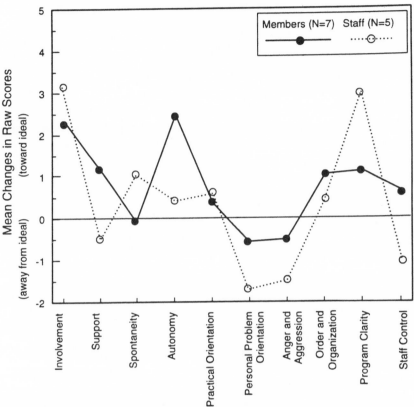

treatment environment cannot be changed toward a static ideal. Feed-back may promote changes in preferences as well as in the actual treatment environment.

An ongoing formative evaluation can help to make programs more responsive to their members and to teach them problem-solving skills. For example, Shinn, Perkins, and Cherniss (1980) provided feedback about the treatment environment to facilitate program development in six residential programs for youth; six other programs served as a comparison group. Staff perceptions of the treatment climate improved over time in the experimental programs, compared with their own baselines and with comparison programs. The process was most successful in stable programs in which staff members had control over important decisions. More experienced consultants and longer, more intensive interventions that focused explicitly on developing staff members' problem solving and goal setting skills also facilitated more positive outcomes (see also Shinn, 1982). (For other examples of the use of COPES to help improve programs, see Friedman, 1982; Friedman, Jeger, and Slotnik, 1982.)

Key Aspects of the Assessment and Feedback Process

The data-based feedback process we have described is the essence of formative program evaluation. The social climate measures are easy to administer, and the process does not require technically trained evaluators. The process is especially effective in small, stable settings in which participants interact frequently and can exert control over at least some aspects of the intervention program.

In essence, program evaluators and consultants can use the WAS and COPES to measure a program's treatment climate, give feedback, and plan interventions. The scales encourage residents and staff to think about their program along 10 meaningful dimensions, each of which can be changed. The resulting information can guide residents' and staff members' efforts to improve their program, focus these efforts on a few well-defined areas, lessen the chance of conflicting goals, and make effective change more likely. Moreover, systemic feedback about the treatment environment provides an opportunity for managers and staff to consider their impact on the program and on clients' satisfaction and self-confidence.

After firsthand experience with formative evaluation, clients and program personnel may be more receptive to subsequent research, including an assessment of the determinants of the program's treatment climate and it's impact on clients' treatment outcome. Before focusing on these issues, we turn to the use of the COPES in assessing program implementation and comparing programs.

7

Assessing the Implementation of Community Programs

As we described earlier (chapter 4), program evaluators need to obtain systematic information to ensure that a program is adequately implemented. Without such information, evaluators may unwittingly compare programs that do not differ as intended or examine outcomes of programs that do not in fact have an active, integrated treatment environment. To review, there are three main sets of standard for program implementation: normative data on conditions in other programs, which allow the evaluator to see how one program compares with others; specifications of an ideal treatment program; and theoretical analysis or expert judgment (Sechrest et al., 1979). To illustrate these standards for community programs, we describe implementation assessments of alcoholism and drug treatment programs, of the generalization of a treatment model from the program to the group level, and of psychiatric and dual diagnosis programs.

Assessing Program Implementation

Alcoholism Treatment Programs

To prepare for a comparative outcome evaluation, we applied the COPES to five residential alcoholism programs, including Pathways, the halfway house program described in chapter 6, a Salvation Army program, a public county-funded program, a private, for-profit, aversion conditioning program, and a private, for-profit, milieu-oriented program (Moos et al., 1990). To illustrate the assessment of treatment implementation, we describe four of these programs here. (For the COPES profile of the halfway house, see figure 6.3.)

The Salvation Army and public, county-funded programs. Figure 7.1 shows the COPES profiles for residents in the Salvation Army and public, county-funded programs. Although the residents in these two programs were similar, the treatment environments were quite different. Residents in both programs saw involvement and spontaneity as above average compared with normative data. Salvation Army residents reported more involvement than county-funded clients did. Residents in the Salvation Army program also reported above average emphasis on support, while county-funded clients did not.

With respect to treatment orientation, residents in both programs appraised independence, concern about personal problems, and the open expression of anger as somewhat above the norm. Salvation Army residents were strongly encouraged to develop practical skills to assist them to adapt to life in the community, but the county-funded program had somewhat below average emphasis on this area.

There were some differences in the perceived structure of the programs. Salvation Army clients saw their program as clear and well organized, whereas this was not true in the county-funded program. This latter finding is consistent with the constant rescheduling of activities and meetings that we observed in the county-funded program. Residents in both programs saw staff control as about average.

Overall, there are some sharp contrasts between these two programs. The Salvation Army program encouraged clients and staff to interact with and support one another. The program emphasized community living skills as exemplified by its training school and the importance given to learning vocational skills. The Salvation Army program was also well organized and clear in its expectations. In contrast, the county-funded program was just average on support and was below average on practical orientation and organization.

The aversion conditioning program. Figure 7.2 shows the COPES profiles for the aversion conditioning program. Residents and staff agreed closely in their perceptions of the treatment climate. Both groups reported high support and spontaneity but little autonomy, which is consistent with the structured schedule patients followed during their two-week stay. Although there was little focus on practical orientation or the expression of anger, residents were encouraged to try to understand their personal problems.

FIGURE 7.1
COPES Form R Profiles for the Salvation Army and
Public County-Funded Programs

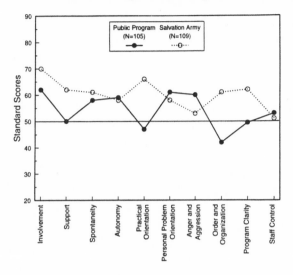

FIGURE 7.2
COPES Form R Profiles for the Aversion Conditioning Program

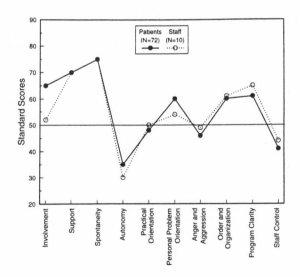

The structured treatment schedule is reflected in the emphasis on organization and clarity. At the same time, there was little reliance on staff control. Thus, the aversion conditioning program was highly structured, but nevertheless encouraged residents to feel involved and to share their personal problems.

The milieu-oriented program. As part of the implementation analysis, we obtained COPES data from a sample of residents and staff in each program to provide initial feedback and elicit cooperation in the evaluation. At that time, the milieu-oriented program was about to undergo a series of changes. This program initially had relied on films and lectures to reeducate clients with substance abuse problems. Residents spent a great deal of time in their rooms, wore pajamas all day, and had their meals brought to their rooms. Although residents socialized informally, group therapy sessions were not included in the treatment regimen.

Concurrent with the beginning of our project, the program hired a new director who established a therapeutic milieu and family-type atmosphere. Television sets were removed from residents' rooms, and family-style meals were served in the dining room. Residents stopped wearing pajamas during the day, were assigned light housekeeping duties, began organizing their own film and discussion sessions, and gave personal care and attention to incoming residents. Several types of group treatment were initiated. An alumni organization was started by an active group of recovered graduates of the program to help current residents plan for their life after discharge.

Figure 7.3 shows COPES profiles based on residents' perceptions before and after these changes. On the whole, residents were more positive about the program after the changes were made. Residents' involvement increased dramatically, probably because of the new director's effort to get residents invested in program activities. The alumni's efforts to explain the value of the program are reflected in heightened practical orientation and program clarity. Thus, the COPES profiles clearly reflected the changes the new director instituted. Moreover, the breadth of the innovations was shown by a positive change in nine of the ten dimensions.

Comparing the programs. The COPES profiles, which distinguish the programs in ways that are consistent with their treatment orientations, complement the information we obtained on treatment quantity. For example, they show that required participation in treatment activi-

FIGURE 7.3
COPES Form R Profiles for the Milieu-Oriented Program

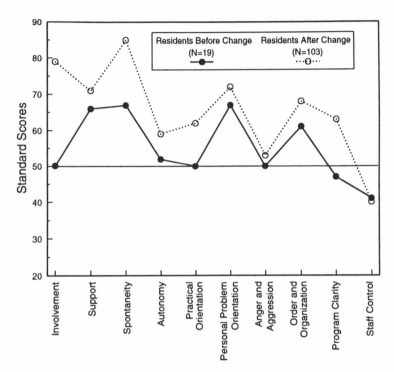

ties does not ensure a highly supportive treatment environment; patients in the county-funded program participated in a variety of meetings and program activities, but the emphasis on support, as tapped by the COPES, was just average. By contrast, the revamped milieu-oriented program, which maintained an even more active schedule for clients, was substantially above the norm on all three relationship dimensions.

The profiles also reveal that an adequate amount of treatment does not necessarily ensure positive treatment quality. Treatment climate may be only moderately associated with the intensity of treatment, the professional background of the staff, and the staffing level. In spite of their active schedule for residents and similar high staff-resident ratio and staff training, the county-funded program lacked organization and clarity, whereas the milieu-oriented program was above average on these system maintenance dimensions after the program changes were made.

Conversely, programs that are brief and use very few treatment components can create a positive climate. The aversion conditioning program is a case in point; although the program emphasized the use of conditioning procedures and medications almost to the exclusion of other treatment components, residents and staff reported good interpersonal relationships and some orientation toward discussing personal problems. These qualities may enhance the effectiveness of behaviorally oriented treatment programs. This program also demonstrates that structure is compatible with good interpersonal relationships and the open expression of anger.

A program run by nonmedical staff can develop a very positive social climate, as the Salvation Army program demonstrates. Paraprofessional staff can establish relationships with clients that are just as empathic and helpful as those established by highly trained professionals (Hattie, Sharpley, and Rogers, 1984). As noted later in this chapter, programs with and without professionally trained staff did not differ on the three relationship dimensions, although the programs without professional staff had somewhat less focus on personal growth. Results for the Salvation Army are consistent with this pattern, as are AA meetings, which typically are highly involving, supportive, expressive, and structured, although chaired by recovering alcoholic individuals who typically do not have professional mental health training (Montgomery, Miller, and Tonigan, 1993).

Overall, the clients in these programs apparently developed a unique camaraderie—an interest in sharing experiences and helping each other—that may be facilitated by their shared problem of alcoholism. Such support is not typical of most psychiatric programs, to which clients are admitted for a variety of reasons. The relatively rich staffing in the alcoholism programs also may help to promote a more positive treatment environment.

Our implementation analysis showed us that we were examining a set of active and varied alcoholism programs. Thus, we proceeded with an impact evaluation (Moos et al., 1990). In addition to its value as a precursor to an outcome study, treatment implementation assessment can detect a short-term deterioration in treatment quantity or quality. If a program is found to be inadequately implemented in either regard, staff can make efforts to improve it.

FIGURE 7.4
COPES Form R Profiles for Residents and Staff in Second Genesis Programs (from Bell, 1983)

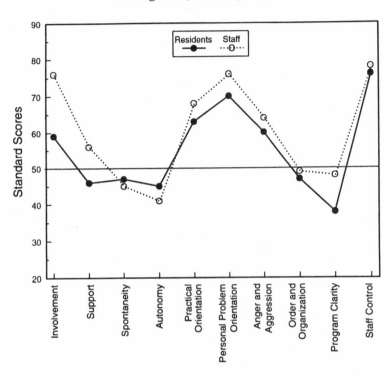

Drug Treatment Programs

One potentially effective way to treat individuals with severe drug abuse problems is to establish a residential therapeutic community (TC) program based on the Synanon, Phoenix House, Day Top, or Second Genesis models. In general, such programs attempt to develop a highly structured and expressive milieu in which clients can enhance their work and social skills and try to understand the reasons for their substance abuse and psychological problems. Following these ideas, Bell (1983) examined the implementation of three Second Genesis TC programs composed of young adult clients, almost all of whom had severe drug abuse problems and prior criminal justice convictions.

As shown in figure 7.4, residents saw these programs as moderately involving, oriented toward the development of social and work skills, self-understanding, and the open expression of anger, and highly structured. Unexpectedly, support and spontaneity were lacking, there was little emphasis on self-direction, and the programs were neither clear nor well organized. In general, staff agreed with residents' perceptions, although they saw the programs as somewhat more involving, supportive, and clear.

According to Bell (1983), the structured work program and activity schedule created a sense of community, but staff members' attempts to avoid the possibility of being manipulated by developing close relationships with clients contributed to the lack of support. An emphasis on businesslike and respectful relationships between residents and staff members and the need to control residents' impulsive behavior contributed to the lack of spontaneity; the expression of affect was encouraged only in scheduled psychotherapy groups.

Second Genesis programs emphasize both practical and personal problem orientation. Residents follow a daily work schedule, learn practical self-care and social skills, and focus on making detailed plans to find employment and develop a drug-free life style after discharge. Rehabilitation counselors facilitate these goals and part-time teachers offer on-site educational activities. With respect to self-disclosure, psychotherapy groups provide a structured framework within which residents share personal experiences and try to understand and thereby control their behavior.

Although these programs are highly structured and have explicit rules and sanctions, residents do not have a clear idea about their individual treatment plans and they report inconsistent application of program rules. In part, Second Genesis' policy of ongoing program change causes substantial day-to-day uncertainty. More profoundly, however, residents' uncertainty about the program may contribute to a lack of trust in staff members' actions and decisions. Another contributing factor may be the somewhat conflicting demands for residents' independence and leadership in the context of a highly structured program in which residents cannot question the staff's authority.

There is an underlying dilemma in residential substance abuse treatment: how to create an environment that incorporates both freedom and structure. Structure is needed to control residents' substance use as well as their impulsive and aggressive behavior; at the same time, freedom and openness are needed to promote residents' self-exploration and expression of affect and ultimately their self-reliance. To examine this issue with respect to individuals' preferences, Penk and Robinowitz (1978) assessed substance abuse clients' actual and preferred treatment program.

Clients saw their program as moderately expressive and oriented toward self-understanding, and, at the same time, as relatively structured, especially in terms of high staff control. Clients wanted the program to place much more emphasis on expressiveness, as well as on involvement, support, and practical orientation. In general, the staff agreed with the clients' perceptions and preferences. In contrast, psychiatric patients in a comparison program felt that they did not need as much focus on expressiveness and staff felt that they did not need as much focus on control. These findings support the idea that well-implemented substance abuse programs should promote clients' expressiveness within a relatively structured environment.

Implementation of a Program Treatment Model at the Group Level

A residential program may have an underlying treatment model and establish am overall environment consistent with that model. One important question is whether the mutual support and psychotherapy groups in the program accurately reflect the program's underlying philosophy. To focus on this issue, Moffett (1991) used the COPES to describe the social climate of Satori, a TC for substance-dependent clients, and the Group Environment Scale (GES; Moos, 1994a) to describe three psychotherapy groups within the community. These assessments were made on seventeen occasions over a ten-year interval.

The Satori program was designed as a highly structured TC oriented toward residents with personality disorders. It involved an extensive set of rules and a strong practical orientation as reflected by an emphasis on learning daily living skills and participation in part-time paid work. The program tried to facilitate residents' understanding of the causes of substance abuse while at the same time controlling their substance use and coping with their impulsivity and aggression.

The Satori community. Residents described the Satori program's social climate as quite consistent with the underlying treatment philosophy. Compared with normative data, the program was somewhat above average in involvement and spontaneity; oriented strongly toward learning practical skills, self-disclosure, and the open expression of anger; and relatively high in staff control. Strikingly, Satori's social climate was relatively stable over a ten-year period. It reflected a differentiated and well-implemented treatment approach. As intended by its designers, Satori was somewhat more structured than a normative therapeutic community.

Satori's psychotherapy groups. Satori residents described the social climate of each of the program's three psychotherapy groups quite similarly, indicating consistent implementation of the treatment philosophy. All three groups were task-focused and oriented toward self-discovery and the open expression of anger. They also were above the average of normative psychotherapy and mutual support groups on cohesion and leader support, as well as on organization and leader control. However, they were seen as less innovative.

The social climate of the overall program and the program's component psychotherapy groups was similar in its orientation toward practical problem solving and learning task-related skills, self-discovery, the open expression of anger, and staff or leader control. These findings indicate that an overall treatment program and psychotherapy groups in that program can be implemented in a stable and consistent way.

Psychiatric and Dual Diagnosis Programs

We have seen that community-based substance abuse programs can have active, well-implemented treatment environments. The programs we studied had a cadre of experienced staff with specialized training in substance abuse treatment and had relatively cognitively intact patients with a common type of disorder. In contrast, in community programs for psychiatric and dually diagnosed clients (that is, individuals with more than one psychiatric disorder or with both a psychiatric and a substance abuse disorder), clients are typically more severely disturbed and staff may be less likely to have specialized training. The treatment models for these types of patients also are less well developed (Swindle et al., 1995). Nevertheless, many of these programs are quite well implemented.

Psychiatric versus substance abuse programs. In a project that focused on both psychiatric and substance abuse programs, Timko (1995) obtained COPES data on sixty-two community programs; a total of twenty-three were primarily for psychiatric patients and thirty-nine were primarily for substance abuse patients. According to both clients' and staff members' reports, on average the psychiatric programs were characterized by less involvement and support, less focus on self-direction, skills development, and self-understanding, and less organization and staff control. These differences also held for hospital programs. Accordingly, programs for psychiatric patients appear to have less well developed and conceptually integrated treatment environments than do programs for substance abuse patients.

Group home and day hospital programs. To focus further on this issue, Manning (1989) assessed six Australian Richmond Fellowship homes for psychiatrically disturbed adults. Consistent with the Fellowship's orientation toward social rehabilitation, residents and staff appraised the programs as well-implemented therapeutic communities, that is, they were seen as expressive and clear and focused on self-direction, skills development, and self-understanding, and as moderate to low on organization and staff control.

Day hospital programs can also develop a therapeutic community milieu. Thus, Comstock et al. (1985) organized an intensive ambulatory care program with therapy groups that emphasized open communication and self-understanding and with a range of skills training and educational activities. As expected, the program placed high emphasis on all three relationship dimensions and on personal problem orientation. There was relatively less emphasis on organization, clarity, and staff control. Importantly, there was a decline in clients' medical and psychiatric health care costs from two years before to two years after participation in the program.

Domiciliaries. The growing tendency to sharply curtail acute patient care has led to the development of hospital-based transitional residential care programs. For example, the VA has a nationwide program of treatment-oriented domiciliaries for homeless veterans, many of whom have substance abuse and psychiatric disorders. Leda et al. (1990) found that these programs are patterned after a structured therapeutic community model and emphasize active treatment and rehabilitation. Clients are encouraged to acquire basic social and vocational skills, to develop a regular daily routine, and, to a lesser extent, to enhance their self-understanding. Staff control is high, which reflects the need for structure among clients in this type of rehabilitation program (see also Leda et al., 1989). However, the programs were not seen as especially supportive, self-directed, clear, or well-organized.

As in the Second Genesis programs Bell (1983) studied, the high level of structure in these domiciliaries may detract somewhat from the development of clients' expressiveness and independence. Accordingly, clients who are treated in community facilities may have better outcomes (Moos, King, and Patterson, 1996).

Supported housing. Traditional supportive housing models emphasize a linear continuum of services whereby a client moves from the most restrictive and intensively staffed setting to less restrictive alternatives. In contrast, supported housing emphasizes the values of consumer choice, independence, participation, ongoing support, and permanence. The supportive housing model forces clients to move when they reach a certain level of functioning, and this disrupts their relationships. The idea behind supported housing is that the individual has a relatively permanent home. Boydell and Everett (1992) evaluated supported housing in a low-rise apartment building comprised of fourteen individual units with additional common space for collective activities.

Clients and staff saw the housing environment as above average in the quality of client-staff relationships and in autonomy and practical and personal problem orientation, and low in staff control. At a follow-up assessment one year later, clients reported increases in practical and personal problem orientation; staff reported increases in practical orientation and organization. Overall, the supported housing project was well implemented in terms of its social climate.

Programs with Professional versus Paraprofessional Staff

As noted earlier, programs with paraprofessional staff may be very well implemented with respect to their treatment environment. To examine this issue in more depth, we compared thirty-two programs that had professionally trained staff members, such as psychiatrists, psychologists, and social workers, with twenty-two programs that had only paraprofessional staff. The clients in the two sets of programs were comparable. The two groups of programs were equally well implemented in the three relationship areas, especially involvement and support (figure 7.5). However, programs with professionally trained staff placed more emphasis on all four personal growth areas, especially practical and personal problem orientation. In contrast, programs with paraprofessional staff placed more emphasis on all three system maintenance dimensions.

FIGURE 7.5
COPES Form R Profiles for Clients in Programs with Professional or Paraprofessional Staff

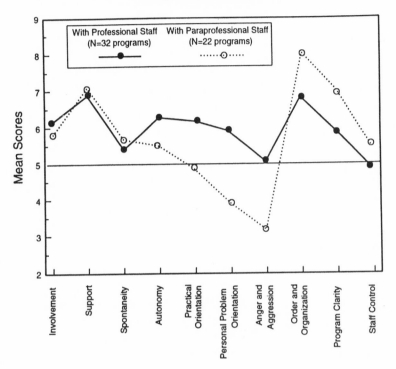

To understand these differences in more detail, we compared clients' responses to specific COPES items. Items on the personal growth dimensions on which clients in programs with professionally trained staff answered true more often include: "Members are taught specific new skills in this program" and "Members are expected to make detailed specific plans for the future." Clients in these programs were more likely to answer false to the following items: "There is relatively little emphasis on teaching members solutions to practical problems," "There is relatively little discussion about exactly what members will be doing after they leave the program," and "Members are rarely encouraged to discuss their personal problems here."

On the system maintenance dimensions, clients in programs with professionally trained staff answered true more often to the following items: "Things are sometimes very disorganized around here"; "The day room or living room is often untidy"; and "People are always changing their minds here." Items on which clients in these programs answered false more often include: "The staff make sure that this place is always neat"; "It is important to carefully follow the program rules here"; and "The staff make and enforce all the rules here."

These findings show that the presence of professionally trained staff increases emphasis on the personal growth dimensions, in that the program is more likely to focus on self-direction, the development of work and social skills, self-understanding, and the open expression of anger. In contrast, paraprofessional staff emphasize organization, clarity, and control somewhat more than professionally trained staff do.

The high quality of personal relationships in programs with paraprofessional staff is consistent with the idea that the quality of relationships between clients and staff is independent of the level of staff members' professional training. With respect to the system maintenance dimensions, professionally trained staff may play down these areas somewhat because of their concern that too much structure may stifle clients' independence.

Overall, the findings imply that professionally trained staff should be encouraged to place more emphasis on program structure, while paraprofessional staff should be educated to enhance independence and practical problem-solving skills. The generational shift we identified toward more staff control in community programs (chapter 5) shows that structure is valued more highly now than it was in the past. Moreover, there has been a substantial increase in well-trained paraprofessional staff, such as certified alcohol and drug counselors, who do promote more emphasis on the personal growth areas (chapter 8).

A Typology of Community Programs

Earlier we identified six types of hospital programs and noted how such a typology can be used to compare programs and to examine the adequacy of program implementation (chapter 4). To identify types of community programs and examine their resemblance to hospital programs, we conducted a cluster analysis of COPES data based on residents' perceptions of 78 programs in the United States and the United Kingdom (UK). In fact, we identified six types of community programs that are closely comparable to the six types of hospital programs.

FIGURE 7.6
**COPES Form R Profiles for Residents in Therapeutic Community
and Relationship-Oriented Programs**

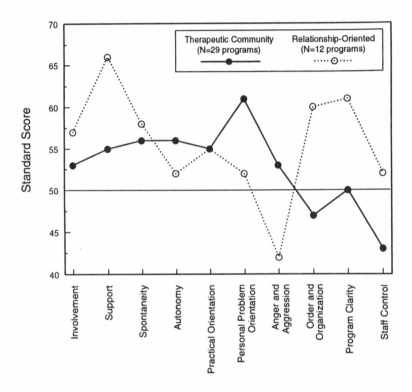

Therapeutic Community and Relationship-Oriented Programs

The first cluster of therapeutic community (TC) programs consists
of twenty-nine of the seventy-eight programs. These programs, shown
in figure 7.6, are moderately supportive and expressive. In addition,
they have high performance expectations; that is, they focus on all
four of the personal growth areas, especially self-direction and self-
understanding. Similar to the hospital-based TC programs, these community programs are relatively low on all three of the system maintenance dimensions. This cluster includes twenty American programs
and nine programs in the UK; of the American programs, fourteen are
well-staffed day-care or day treatment programs and only three are
community care homes.

FIGURE 7.7
COPES Form R Profiles for Residents in Action-Oriented
and Insight-Oriented Programs

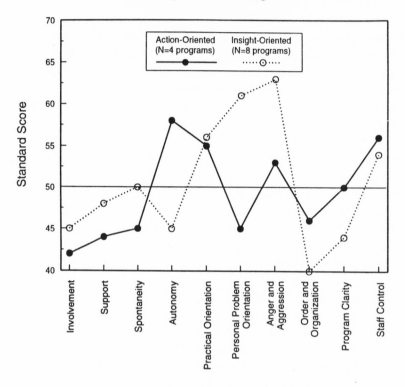

Figure 7.6 also shows the profile of the twelve relationship-oriented programs. These programs emphasize supportive and open interpersonal relationships in conjunction with the development of clear expectations in the context of a well-organized and structured setting. These programs have fewer performance expectations than the TC programs; they have moderate emphasis on autonomy and practical and personal problem orientation and discourage the expression of anger. Nine of the programs are American; six of these are either halfway houses or community care homes.

Action-Oriented and Insight-Oriented Programs

The four action-oriented programs emphasize residents' self-direction and the development of work and social skills in a moderately controlled setting (figure 7.7). In general, they lack the support, organization, and explicit policies needed to effectively foster these expectations for clients' performance.

The eight insight-oriented programs, also shown in figure 7.7, value self-understanding and the open expression of anger in the context of moderate emphasis on social and vocational training. Surprisingly, however, they do not emphasize the development of supportive interpersonal relationships, nor do they attempt to promote residents' self direction. Moreover, although staff control is elevated, there is very little emphasis on organization or clarity.

Action-oriented and insight-oriented programs are somewhat complementary. Action-oriented programs are high on self-direction but play down self-understanding and the expression of anger, whereas insight-oriented programs are high on self-understanding and the expression of anger but low on self-direction. Even though both sets of programs emphasize the development of work and social skills, the poor quality of relationships and lack of organization and clarity do not bode well for these programs' clients.

Control-Oriented and Undifferentiated Programs

Unexpectedly, almost 25 percent of the community programs fell into a control-oriented cluster. As shown in figure 7.8, these programs do not emphasize either the development of supportive relationships or performance expectations associated with any of the personal growth goals. Staff and caretakers are oriented primarily toward maintaining a well-organized and highly-structured milieu. Most surprisingly, five of the seventeen American programs in this cluster are designated vocational and rehabilitation workshops. Ten programs are community care homes for veterans and two are VA-affiliated day-care centers. Most of the programs serve somewhat older, more chronic clients who may need a relatively high degree of structure and less intense interpersonal relationships.

The six undifferentiated programs are well below average in all areas except the expression of anger and aggression and staff control (figure 7.8). These programs try to manage acutely disturbed patients in an open community setting and thus seek to institute more control than most other community programs. However, these programs are unusually low in organization and clarity and have not developed

FIGURE 7.8
**COPES Form R Profiles for Residents in Control-Oriented
and Undifferentiated Programs**

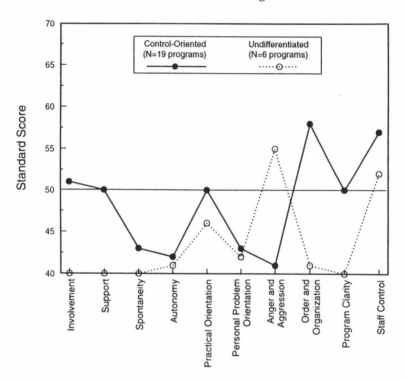

supportive interpersonal relationships or an emphasis on personal
growth goals.

The Variability of Community Programs

The findings highlight considerable diversity in the treatment environments of community programs. Similarly, on the basis of a cluster
analysis of COPES data on forty-nine facilities, Downs and Fox (1993)
identified four distinct types of community homes for chronically mentally ill adults. These types varied primarily in their levels of support,
structure, and performance expectations.

Together with our work on hospital programs (chapter 4), these
findings show that the quality of the treatment milieu cannot be in-

ferred simply from knowledge about the location or type of facility. Control-oriented community care settings provide less treatment and less impetus toward personal growth goals than hospital-based therapeutic community programs do. Moreover, some community facilities are strongly oriented toward the development of social and vocational skills, whereas others have little if any treatment orientation. These conclusions hold even though current community programs are much more treatment oriented than was the case twenty years ago.

Community versus Hospital Programs

An emphasis on reducing health care costs has led to a sharp decline in the length of acute inpatient care and intensive pressure to identify alternative, less expensive forms of care. At the same time, many patients now have much more severe and chronic disorders than a decade ago, and a much larger proportion of patients have more than one psychiatric diagnosis and/or comorbid substance abuse diagnoses. Accordingly, there is growing interest in developing new forms of community care for severely disturbed clients and in comparing the quality of treatment in community and hospital programs (for example, see Geller, 1991; Leff et al., 1996; Walz and Goldstein, 1992).

Psychiatric patients often enter the hospital when they are acutely disturbed and in a severe crisis situation. With intensive inpatient treatment, many of these patients show substantial short-term improvement and then are discharged to a community facility. Accordingly, compared with hospital programs, community programs for psychiatric patients should have a more active and integrated treatment milieu.

A comparison of fifteen hospital and twenty-three community psychiatric programs based on Timko's (1995) data supported these ideas. On average, according to staff members' reports, the community programs were more supportive and expressive, more oriented toward self-direction, and clearer and better organized. In contrast, the hospital programs were higher on anger and aggression. Clients also appraised community programs as clearer and more expressive and self-directed.

In general, these findings held for substance abuse programs, although the differences were less extensive. Compared with hospital programs (N=11), staff members' saw community substance abuse programs (N=39) as more supportive and expressive and as better organized and higher on staff control. Clients saw them only as more expressive. Similarly, Wilson (1993) found that freestanding substance abuse programs were somewhat higher on involvement and the open expression of anger than were hospital programs. However, because these differences were relatively small, Wilson concluded that facility location did not substantially influence treatment climate.

These findings imply that, on average, community programs are somewhat more supportive, directed, and structured than are hospital programs. This is a change from the situation in the past, when many community programs were newly developed and relatively poorly staffed, and provided few if any treatment services. As proponents of deinstitutionalization planned more than 40 years ago, the locus of active treatment seems finally to be moving from the hospital to the community.

Group Homes for Acute Schizophrenic Clients

One important question is whether individuals with acute schizophrenic disorders can be treated in a community rather than a hospital setting. To examine this issue, Mosher and his colleagues (Mosher, 1991; Mosher and Menn, 1978; Mosher, Menn, and Matthews, 1975; Wendt et al., 1983) developed Soteria House (*Soteria* is the word for deliverance in Greek), a program rooted in the tradition of intensive interpersonal intervention, the concepts of moral treatment, and crisis theory. They compared two matched cohorts of first-admission, unmarried, schizophrenic clients between fifteen and thirty years of age who were judged to be in need of hospitalization.

Soteria House accommodated six residents at a time; there were six nonprofessional staff members, two of whom were on duty at any one time. Staff had few performance expectations of residents and there was a minimum of organized structure. In contrast, the comparison inpatient program was a well-staffed (1.5 staff members per patient), active treatment facility oriented toward crisis intervention and the use of high doses of medication. The program provided individual therapy, a crisis group and other group treatment, a couple's group, occupational therapy, and a daily community meeting.

Compared with the inpatient unit, which was assessed with the WAS, Soteria House residents and staff saw their program as more supportive and expressive and oriented more toward autonomy, self-understanding, and the open expression of anger. However, Soteria was well below average in practical orientation and in all three of the system maintenance dimensions. In contrast to the situation on the inpatient unit, residents and staff saw Soteria as quite close to their preferred program. These patterns, which remained quite stable over a four-year interval, are consistent with the differences in the two programs' treatment orientations.

Initial six-month and one-year outcome data showed that individuals treated in Soteria had less psychopathology and were more likely to be working full-time and to be living alone or with peers (rather than with parents or other relatives). Soteria's treatment philosophy and longer treatment duration (an average of 167 days versus twenty-one days in the hospital program) facilitated the transition from a family-based to a peer-based social network, which may be associated with more self-direction and better long-term outcome.

Even though it focused on young, acutely disturbed schizophrenic patients who are especially in need of support and self-understanding, Soteria's relative lack of practical orientation and structure may be problematic. To examine another residential alternative to hospitalization, Mosher et al. (1986) compared Soteria with Crossing Place, a program for older, long term, mentally ill patients. Crossing Place emphasized practical orientation more strongly than Soteria did; it was also better organized and higher on staff control. Crossing Place was especially well implemented: it combined support and self-understanding with the focus on skills development and structure that many chronic patients need.

Partial Care Programs

Partial care programs can be provided either in hospital or community settings. In this vein, Luft and Fakhouri (1979) described a hospital-based day care program that combined occupational therapy and recreational activities with daily group counseling. An alternative community-based program placed more emphasis on structured social experiences, leisure time planning, and community involvement and discouraged clients' discussion of their symptoms and past problems. The hospital program met five days each week and the community program met twice each week.

Compared with the hospital program, clients and staff saw the com-

munity program as more supportive, spontaneous, and practically oriented, and as more structured; in contrast, the hospital program was
oriented more toward self-understanding and the expression of anger.
Overall, the hospital program was more intensive and insight-oriented,
whereas the community program was more supportive and oriented
toward skills training. Both partial care programs were associated with
reduced inpatient episodes and days, but the community program cost
much less.

Community Mental Health Center versus General Hospital Programs

A major legislative reform in psychiatric treatment in Italy involved
closing admissions to mental hospitals and developing psychiatric units
in general hospitals and alternative community mental health services.
A key aspect of the rationale was to democratize the locus and environment of care as part of a broader social reform. In fact, compulsory
admissions and the number of psychiatric patients in mental hospitals
declined sharply, but the overall rate of inpatient psychiatric care remained stable because of increased admissions to general hospitals
(Mosher and Burti, 1989).

Burti, Glick, and Tansella (1990) used Italian versions of the COPES
and the WAS to compare a psychiatric unit in a general hospital with a
community mental health center run by the same staff. The idea was to
facilitate continuity of care and long-term supportive services. According to staff, the community center was more involving, supportive, and oriented toward autonomy, but, unexpectedly, less focused on
the development of practical skills and higher on staff control. In the
freer, more open community treatment setting, staff may have experienced a need for more control in order to provide clients with an
appropriate structure for their daily activities. More generally, however, both the hospital and community treatment programs were implemented in line with the new Italian philosophy of more democratic
treatment.

Residential versus Outpatient Programs

There is considerable debate about the relative value of residential
versus outpatient substance abuse programs (Finney, Hahn, and Moos,
1996), but little is known about differences in these programs' treat-

ment environments. When Friedman, Glickman, and Kovach (1986a) addressed this issue in a comparison of twenty-seven residential and thirty outpatient programs for youth, they found that residential programs were more supportive and structured and higher on practical and personal problem orientation and the open expression of anger. These findings held for both clients' and staff members' perceptions; moreover, they held after controlling for clients' demographic characteristics.

Friedman and colleagues (1986a) speculate that these differences may reflect the full-time, live-in nature of residential programs, which encompass much more of the clients' time and have more opportunity to engage clients in treatment. Compared with outpatient programs, residential programs may provide clients not only with a stronger focus on developing self-care and vocational skills, but also with a temporary structured respite during which they can garner their personal resources. In support of this idea, staff in small therapeutic communities reported more order, clarity, and control and rated their programs as more effective than did staff in outpatient methadone maintenance programs (Bausell, Rinkus, and Watson, 1979).

On average, residential programs in the community appear to be as well implemented as are hospital programs. Nevertheless, some community programs are highly restrictive and custodial and some hospital programs are client oriented and have well-motivated staff who are optimistic about clients' performance potential. These findings confirm the conclusion that the location of a program need not determine the quality of its services (Allen, Gillespie, and Hall, 1989; Garety and Morris, 1984; Walz and Goldstein, 1992). More broadly, there is considerable diversity in hospital and community programs' treatment climates. These findings raise a question about the underlying reasons for this diversity, an issue to which we turn next.

Part III

Determinants and Outcomes
of Treatment Environments

8

Determinants of Program Climate

We have seen that hospital and community programs vary widely in the quality of resident and staff relationships, the emphasis on personal growth dimensions such as autonomy and practical orientation, and the level of organization and control. This finding raises important questions: Why do treatment environments develop in such disparate ways? What leads to an emphasis on support, or on autonomy, or on organization and control? In this chapter, we examine four sets of factors that shape treatment environments: the institutional context, physical features, policies and services, and suprapersonal factors or the aggregate characteristics of residents and staff.

Factors that Shape Program Climate

To address this issue, we expanded the conceptual framework shown in figure 1.1 to focus on the connections between panels I and III in the model. As shown in figure 8.1, the institutional context (factors such as ownership, size, and staffing) and the other three sets of environmental factors can directly or indirectly influence the treatment climate (Timko and Moos, 1990). The model posits that the impact of the institutional context and of physical, policy, and resident and staff characteristics stems in part from the treatment environment they help to promote. In turn, the treatment environment can alter the influence of the other four domains on residents' and staff members' morale and well-being.

For example, physical amenities and social-recreational aids, such as a lounge furnished with comfortable chairs, may enhance cohesion

FIGURE 8.1
Determinants of Social Climate in Psychiatric and
Substance Abuse Treatment Programs

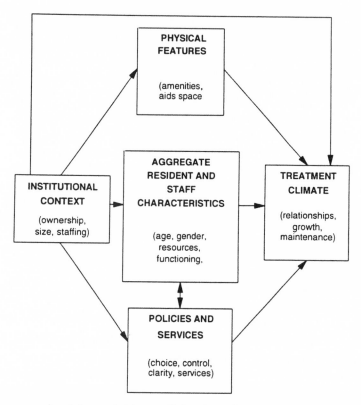

by encouraging joint activities; policies that allow residents more choice in their activities of daily living are likely to contribute to residents' independence. Residents with more cognitive and functional resources are likely to engage in more social interaction and independent activities and thereby promote a sense of cohesion and self-direction.

We use the framework to guide us in focusing on the associations between the institutional context, physical features, policies and services, the aggregate characteristics of residents and staff, and the treatment climate. We examined these associations in the initial samples of hospital and community programs (Moos, 1974), in a more recent sample of psychiatric and substance abuse programs (Timko, 1995; Timko and Moos, 1996), and in a nationwide sample of residential facilities for older adults (Moos and Lemke, 1994). In facilities for older adults, we assessed social climate with the Sheltered Care Environment Scale (SCES), which also measures relationship (cohesion, conflict), personal growth (independence, self-disclosure), and system maintenance (organization) dimensions (Lemke and Moos, 1987; Moos and Lemke, in press). We summarize here some of the findings that have emerged from this body of work and from other investigators' research.

Institutional Context

Ownership

According to Arrington and Haddock (1990), nonprofit psychiatric hospitals offer more social benefits in the areas of access to care, services provided, and staff training than for-profit hospitals do. Compared with for-profit providers, nonprofit mental health service providers devote more staff resources to patient care (Schlesinger and Dorwart, 1984) and provide more services (Culhane and Hadley, 1992). More generally, as Shadish (1989) noted, the shift from public- toward private-sector facilities has not improved the quality of care for chronic mental patients, in part because marketplace incentives motivate managers to house patients as cheaply as possible and because potential protective mechanisms, such as informed consumer choice and government regulation, are ineffective countervailing forces.

Compared with for-profit psychiatric and substance abuse programs, not-for-profit facilities placed more emphasis on the development of residents' social and vocational skills and were better organized (Timko and Moos, 1996). We obtained generally similar findings in facilities for older adults. Compared with proprietary facilities, nonprofit facilities were more cohesive and better organized and emphasized independence and resident influence more strongly. Thus, nonprofit facilities seem to be better organized and to emphasize personal growth more than proprietary facilities do; they may also develop a greater sense of community (Table 8.1). These social climate factors are more consistent with the norms of nonprofit settings where the ethos is one of service to the consumer.

TABLE 8.1
Associations between Institutional Context and Treatment Climate

Institutional Context	Treatment Climate					
	Support	Autonomy	Practical	Personal Problem	Order	Staff Control
Nonprofit Ownership	+	+	++		++	
Smaller Size	++	+		+	+	--
Staffing	+	+		+		-

Note.   ++   Strong positive relationship
　　　　+   Moderate positive relationship
　　　　–   Moderate inverse relationship
　　　– –   Strong inverse relationship

Size

In general, practitioners assume that smaller programs are more cohesive and more likely to foster a climate that promotes personal growth, especially one that permits residents to share their personal problems and feelings. Because of a more manageable range of influences, smaller programs should be clearer and better organized than larger programs. In contrast, large size may create a demand for a custodial, control-oriented atmosphere, which may elicit disruptive behavior that in turn justifies more regimentation.

We focused first on the associations between program size, as reflected by the number of patients, and the treatment environment in hospital programs in the United States and the United Kingdom (UK). Program size varied from seven to 140 patients in the United States sample and from seven to seventy-seven patients in the UK sample (Moos, 1972b; 1974, chapter 6). Consistent with expectations, smaller programs were more supportive and expressive and oriented more toward self-understanding. They were also lower on staff control. These findings were comparable in the United States and UK samples.

We also studied sixteen community programs that had an average of twenty-six clients; the range was from six to forty-three. As predicted, smaller programs had more emphasis on support and self-direction and were lower on staff control (Moos, 1974, chapter 12). According to Segal and Moyles (1979), smaller community facilities were more client-centered whereas larger facilities were more management centered.

Program reorganization sometimes provides a unique opportunity to examine the influence of size on treatment climate. When a psychiatric unit for schizophrenic patients was divided into smaller programs, organization increased and aggression declined (Nissen, 1985). In the converse situation, a residential program was centralized from three small houses to one large facility. As expected, residents and staff saw the larger program as less supportive, less oriented toward autonomy and self-understanding, and less clear and well-organized. This negative impact of larger size became more pronounced over time (Hellman et al., 1985).

Trained and experienced staff may alter the typical negative influence of large size on the treatment milieu. In a study of thirty-five Norwegian programs, Friis (1986b) unexpectedly found that larger size was associated with more clarity and more emphasis on self-understanding and the expression of anger. He concluded that the presence of a more stable staff group in the larger programs helped to develop a more positive social climate. This may explain in part why there were no associations between size and the social climate in our sample of psychiatric and substance abuse programs (Timko and Moos, 1996).

Overall, smaller programs are more supportive and expressive and typically have more emphasis on autonomy and self-understanding (table 8.1). With respect to program structure, smaller programs tend to be less bureaucratic and regimented. However, larger programs may be disorganized, especially when staff withdraw from contact with residents or are overwhelmed by the substantial work demands in such programs. It is also important to recognize that more competent residents or staff can counteract the potential negative influence of large size (Friis, 1986b) and that larger programs sometimes provide residents with more opportunities or self-direction (Moos and Lemke, 1994).

Staffing

Higher staffing is often used as an indicator of better quality care and might be expected to be associated with a more cohesive, self-directed, and well-organized social climate. In fact, we found that better staffed hospital programs in the United States were more supportive and expressive and lower on staff control (table 8.1). These findings were replicated in hospital programs in the UK and in community programs (Moos, 1974, chapters 6 and 12; Moos, 1972c). Similarly, Friis (1986b) found that better staffing was associated with more emphasis on self-direction and self-understanding.

Leda, Rosenheck, and Fontana (1991) focused on staffing in transitional residential programs for homeless veterans. They combined eight of the COPES subscales (all but anger and staff control) to form a Therapeutic Activity (TA) index. Better staffed programs were higher on the TA index, as well as on involvement, autonomy, and practical and personal problem orientation. These findings highlight the importance of enriched staffing for the development of a therapeutic treatment milieu in both hospital and community programs. More broadly, however, the amount of staff-patient interaction is likely to have a stronger influence on the treatment milieu than does the level of staffing per se. Richer staffing sometimes may have little or no impact on the treatment climate (Timko and Moos, 1996), perhaps because a high proportion of staff are minimally trained paraprofessionals or because staff have more meetings and interact primarily with each other.

Physical Features

Although a number of studies have shown that psychiatric programs' physical features can influence patients' behavior (e.g. Devlin, 1992), only a few researchers have examined the relationship between physical features and the treatment environment. One problem has been the lack of a consistent way to measure the key sets of physical features in psychiatric and substance abuse programs. To address this issue, Timko (1996) conceptualized physical features in terms of seven dimensions, four of which we consider here. These dimensions can be measured by the Physical and Architectural Characteristics Inventory (Timko, 1996) in psychiatric and substance abuse programs and by the

Physical and Architectural Features Checklist in congregate facilities for older adults (Moos and Lemke, in press).

Two of the dimensions, physical amenities and social-recreational aids, focus on the presence of physical features that add convenience and comfort to a facility and that foster social and recreational activities. Two other dimensions reflect the allowance of space for resident and staff functions. Space availability is the amount of communal and personal space available to residents. Staff facilities are physical features that make the setting more pleasant for staff; this dimension is important because such features may promote staff morale and contribute to the quality of patient care.

Physical Amenities and Social-Recreational Aids

When psychiatric programs are remodeled, there typically is an increase in physical amenities and social-recreational aids. In one such project, the remodeling added physical amenities that were consistent with the therapeutic orientation: patients' bedrooms were personalized, oak tables replaced metal tables, furniture was arranged in clusters to permit conversation, carpeting replaced vinyl tile floor covering, and pictures and plants were added to communal areas. In general, after these changes were made, involvement, autonomy, and organization increased, especially in the program in which changes had been in place the longest (Corey et al., 1986).

Two other studies have shown that an improvement in physical features can contribute to increased resident involvement and to a better organized program. Specifically, Baldwin (1985) introduced group seating patterns and leisure time resources in unit dayrooms. Residents and staff on the intervention units reported an improvement in the quality of relationships; residents also reported an increase in organization. Christenfeld et al. (1989) also noted that renovation of the physical environment of two psychiatric programs for long-term chronic patients improved staff morale and increased patients' satisfaction with the unit. Table 8.2 summarizes the main findings of these studies.

We obtained comparable findings in residential facilities for older adults. Residents in living groups with more physical amenities and social-recreational aids reported more cohesion, independence, and resident influence. These physical features may enhance cohesion and

TABLE 8.2
Associations between Physical Features, Policies and Services,
and Treatment Climate

Physical and Policy Factors	Treatment Climate					
	Support	Autonomy	Practical	Personal Problem	Order	Staff Control
Physical Features						
Amenities and Social-Recreational Aids	+	+			+	
Space for Residents and Staff	+	+			+	
Policies and Services						
Resident Control	++	++	++	++		
Policy Choice	−	++			−	−
Clarity	+	+	++	++	+	
Health and Treatment Services	+		++	+		

Note. ++ Strong positive relationship
       +   Moderate positive relationship
       −   Moderate inverse relationship
      − − Strong inverse relationship

self-direction because they encourage residents to leave their private quarters to use common areas, and they provide resources with which residents can initiate activities, engage in social interactions, and make productive use of their time (Moos and Lemke, 1994).

Space for Resident and Staff Functions

The findings for space are comparable to those for physical amenities, but they may be specific to congregate residences for older adults. When more space is available for resident functions, residents report more cohesion, more resident influence, and better organization (table 8.2). In congregate residences, the availability of separate areas and adequate space for diverse functions may not only encourage relationships by giving residents the opportunity to join others in preferred activities, but also reduce potential sources of conflict. Adequate space may reduce the tendency to restrict residents through rules and regulations and enable residents to regulate their interpersonal contact, thus giving them a greater feeling of control. Adequate space also facilitates planning and conducting activities, thus contributing to the facility's efficient management (Moos and Lemke, 1994).

Where more space is available for staff, residents view the social climate as more cohesive and as higher on independence and resident influence. Residents see staff as being more available and supportive, in spite of the fact that staff may spend less time in actual proximity to residents. By providing a respite from caregiving responsibilities, facilities for staff may improve staff morale and allow staff to be more supportive in their interactions with residents. When staff members are not in constant physical proximity to residents, they may do more to encourage resident independence and may interfere less with residents' activities. Having space of their own, staff may be more willing to cede control of other areas of the facility to residents.

Policies and Services

Although there has been longstanding interest in psychiatric and substance abuse programs' policies and services, the salient aspects of these domains have only recently been measured systematically. Specifically, Timko (1995) developed the Policy and Services Characteristics Inventory, which measures several important aspects of program policies and services, four of which we consider here: formal institutional structures giving residents potential influence in the facility (resident control), the latitude of choice residents have to establish their own daily routine (policy choice), formal arrangements for communicating about policies and programs (policy clarity), and the availability of health and treatment services in the facility. In congregate facilities for older adults, these dimensions can be measured by the Policy and Program Information Form (Moos and Lemke, in press).

Resident Control and Choice

Policies that enable residents to participate more in the governance of psychiatric and substance abuse programs help to establish a more supportive, self-directed treatment climate that encourages residents' self-understanding and skills development (Timko and Moos, 1996). We obtained similar findings in facilities for older adults. Thus residents' participation in setting policies serves a relationship as well as a task function: it strengthens relationships among residents and staff and gives residents a voice in decisions (table 8.2).

A closely related aspect of program policy is the emphasis on adult status, that is, the extent to which patients are allowed to maintain their independence and dignity, in part by having some choice over their patterns of daily living. According to our findings, hospital programs that allowed patients more choice were higher on autonomy and lower on staff control (Moos, 1974, chapter 6). In facilities for older adults, more choice was also associated with more independence and less staff control.

Staff members sometimes express the fear that individualizing care routines will lead to confusion and inefficiency and that residents who exercise autonomy may disrupt orderly routines and procedures. This was not the case in our initial sample of hospital programs or in facilities for older adults. In the more recent sample of psychiatric and substance abuse programs, however, policies that broadened clients' freedom of decisionmaking about their activities of daily living were associated with less organization as well as with less support. We also found that clients' choice was associated with less emphasis on practical and personal problem orientation, but this was because programs that provided clients with more choice had fewer treatment services (Timko and Moos, 1996).

When clients participate in the governance of a program, support and self-direction can be enhanced without reducing the level of efficiency or organization. With respect to the daily routine, however, program support and organization may decline when clients are given a choice about whether or not to comply with program schedules, such as when they are allowed to sleep late and skip breakfast. This may also happen when policies do not explicitly discourage activities that may isolate individuals from each other, such as when clients are permitted to have a television set in their room.

Clarity of Policies

Clearer policies may increase predictability for residents and staff and, consequently, their feeling of control; they may also contribute to more efficient program facility operation (table 8.2). In fact, in psychiatric and substance abuse programs, residents report more support and organization in programs with more formal avenues for communicating policies. Formal arrangements may increase group cohesion and structure by clarifying expectations and reducing uncertainty for residents. As with the provision of resident control, residents may use formal mechanisms for relationship as well as for task functions. For example, an orientation program for new residents offers an opportunity to get acquainted as well as to learn the rules and routines.

Clearly stated policies also contribute to a social climate that promotes high performance expectations, especially self-direction, skills development, and self-understanding. By making the environment more predictable, clear policies probably enhance residents' motivation and opportunities for personal growth. In contrast, ambiguous policies may contribute to feelings of helplessness.

Health and Treatment Services

A diverse set of health and treatment services may establish high performance expectations and create opportunities for residents' self-development (table 8.2). Accordingly, residents and staff judge programs with more health and treatment services as oriented more toward the development of social and vocational skills and self-understanding; these programs are also somewhat more supportive. One unexpected side effect of the strong emphasis on performance goals may be less spontaneity. Thus, program-sponsored health and treatment services appear to foster a climate of self-development but also may detract somewhat from the formation of expressive relationships (Timko and Moos, 1996). Programs that have more services may be oriented primarily toward preparing residents for discharge and thus play down the open exchange of feelings.

Aggregate Resident and Staff Characteristics

When individuals come together in a social group, they bring with them their own values, norms, and abilities. Treatment programs draw their members in a nonrandom manner and produce distinctive blends of personal characteristics. The aggregate of the patients' and staff members' attributes—the suprapersonal environment—in part defines the treatment environment that forms in a program.

The characteristics of the individuals in a setting are situational variables in that they partially define relevant aspects of the environment. This approach is reflected in Holland's (1985) theory that people's vocational choices are expressions of their personalities and that occupations can be categorized into six groups, each representing a personality type. Because people in an occupational group share important background characteristics, that is, a dominant vocational preference and similar personalities, the members of the group should respond to situations in similar ways and, in doing so, create a characteristic work climate with distinctive demands, rewards, and opportunities.

The same logic applies to psychiatric treatment programs. For example, a program that is composed primarily of younger, relatively well-functioning substance abuse patients is likely to emphasize active participation in group therapy, discussions about personal problems, and decisionmaking forums to shape program policies. Accordingly, the program will be oriented toward self-direction, self-understanding, and the open expression of anger and will play down staff control. In contrast, a program composed primarily of older, more impaired psychiatric patients is likely to have a less growth-oriented and more structured treatment milieu.

Residents' Characteristics

Surprisingly, only a few researchers have examined the link between residents' characteristics and psychiatric and substance abuse programs' treatment environment. In congregate facilities, however, residents' abilities, personal resources, and typical patterns of behavior help shape the social climate. In general, facilities with more women and more socially privileged and functionally able residents develop more positive social climates (Moos and Lemke, 1994).

Residents' age. Programs with a high proportion of older clients consistently are less supportive and less oriented toward clients' personal growth (table 8.3). Thus, Friis (1986b) noted that Norwegian programs with older patients were less involving and supportive and less oriented toward self-understanding. Friis speculated that these age-related shifts in the treatment environment were consistent with older patients' preferences.

TABLE 8.3
**Associations between Residents' and Staff Members' Characteristics
and Treatment Climate**

Resident and Staff Characteristics	Treatment Climate					
	Support	Autonomy	Practical	Personal Problem	Order	Staff Control
Residents						
Age	– –	– –	– –	– –		– –
% Women	+				+	
Social Resources	++	++		++	+	
Mental Impairment	– –	–	– –	– –	–	+
Staff						
Age			–	– –	+	
% Women	+				+	
Experience and Functioning	+	+	+	++		

Note.   ++   Strong positive relationship
         +   Moderate positive relationship
         –   Moderate inverse relationship
         – – Strong inverse relationship

We basically replicated these findings. Specifically, in psychiatric and substance abuse programs with a higher proportion of late-middle-aged and older clients, clients and staff reported less involvement and less emphasis on all four of the personal growth dimensions, most notably practical and personal problem orientation. These programs also were lower in staff control, perhaps because older clients are less impulsive and thus need less structure. Similarly, Willer and Intagliata (1984) noted that group homes whose residents were primarily older (over age 50) had less emphasis on involvement and practical orientation than did homes whose residents were primarily younger.

Proportion of women residents. We thought that programs with a higher proportion of women residents would have a more supportive and well-organized treatment climate. These expectations did not hold in psychiatric or substance abuse programs. In facilities for older adults, however, those with a higher proportion of women residents are more cohesive and well-organized (table 8.3). Moreover, veterans facilities, which are populated primarily by men, tend to be less cohesive and organized and higher on conflict than are community facilities (Moos and Lemke, 1994). Women may be oriented more toward social relationships than are men. In addition, facilities with a higher proportion of men, such as board-and-care homes and domiciliaries, may draw from a less socially integrated section of the population than do those with a more representative proportion of women residents.

Residents' social resources. In programs in which residents have higher aggregate social resources, residents report more support and expressiveness (table 8.3). Several factors may contribute to the greater harmony and openness in these in settings. More privileged resident groups may experience less distress because their programs have more resources, such as privacy and space. Depending on their social background, residents may have different views of the open expression of feelings; for example, among socially advantaged residents, norms may encourage the sharing of personal experiences. In addition, residents with more social resources may be better able to maintain equal status with staff and to reciprocate staff social interactions; in turn, this ability may lead to higher levels of cohesion (Timko and Moos, 1996).

Programs that house residents with more social resources also place more emphasis on self-direction and self-understanding. These findings may also reflect different norms related to residents' social status. Based on their past experience, residents with more social resources may be more responsive to staff encouragement of independence and self-understanding and more effective in voicing their opinions and concerns. If staff see that residents value and effectively use these opportunities, staff may be more likely to institute and maintain procedures that accommodate resident independence and self-disclosure. In addition, residents with higher social status may retain relatively more power in the relationship with staff members than do residents with lower social status.

Residents' mental impairment and diagnoses. Residents' mental impairment and diagnoses are often perceived as major constraints on the treatment climate. Consistent with this idea, programs with more mentally impaired residents were less supportive and well-organized and less oriented toward skills development and self-understanding (Timko and Moos, 1996). Moreover, programs with a higher proportion of psychotic patients were less involving and supportive and less oriented toward autonomy and practical and personal problem orientation; they were also higher on staff control (Friis, 1986b).

Staff Characteristics

Staff members' age. Our findings for staff members' age are conceptually comparable to those for patients' age, perhaps in part because programs with older staff members are more likely to also have older clients. Specifically, psychiatric and substance abuse programs with older staff members tended to have less emphasis on practical and personal problem orientation; however they were no less supportive (table 8.3). In facilities for older adults, staff reported less conflict in settings where more of the staff were over age fifty.

A more mature staff, who are likely to have more work experience, should contribute to predictability and efficiency in a facility. In fact, according to staff in psychiatric and substance abuse programs, a higher proportion of employees over age 50 contributed to better organization. We obtained the same finding in facilities for older adults.

Proportion of women staff. Generalizing from our results on the gender composition of the resident population, we might expect that programs with a higher proportion of women staff members would emphasize interpersonal relationships and organization. In support of this idea, a forensic hospital program with more women staff members was more supportive, and clearer and better organized than was a program with fewer women staff (Goldmeier and Silver, 1988). There also was less anger in the program with more women staff. Similarly, residents view facilities for older adults with more women staff as having less conflict. Again, however, these findings did not hold in psychiatric or substance abuse programs. Overall, the presence of more women staff may exert some influence to enhance interpersonal relationships and program structure (table 8.3).

Staff experience and functioning. More staff experience and better staff functioning are expected to promote a more self-directed, as well as a more supportive and better organized environment (table 8.3). Thus, we found that a higher proportion of college educated staff was associated with more autonomy (Moos, 1974; chapter 12) and that better functioning staff developed more supportive treatment environments that were oriented more toward self-direction and self-understanding (Timko and Moos, 1996). Similarly, Friis (1986b) noted that programs with a higher proportion of well-trained staff were oriented more toward self-understanding; they were also more supportive and lower on staff control.

Our findings in community programs suggest that staff professionalism may be associated specifically with strengthening expectations for residents' performance (chapter 7). However, some paraprofessional staff, such as alcohol and drug counselors, also help to create a strong emphasis on practical and personal problem orientation. Such staff members are well-trained in counseling procedures and many are recovering individuals who can draw on their personal experiences in treatment. This combination of factors may enable them to create a treatment milieu in which clients feel free to discuss personal issues and can learn how to manage practical problems that arise in community living (Timko and Moos, 1996).

Interventions to Improve Treatment Climate

Overall, these findings support the conceptual model and point to some important determinants of the treatment climate. In general, smaller, better staffed, and nonprofit programs are more supportive and expressive and more likely to emphasize clients' self-direction and self-understanding. The presence of more physical amenities and space, and clearer policies that encourage residents' self-direction is also associated with these aspects of the treatment climate. More health and treatment services seem to specifically enhance the emphasis on residents' skills development and self-understanding.

Suprapersonal factors, especially residents' social resources and mental functioning and the presence of younger residents and staff, also promote supportive treatment environments that have higher expectations for residents' performance. More experienced and better trained staff may be especially important in raising the emphasis on clients' personal growth; well-trained paraprofessional staff also contribute to these areas and to program support. Thus, the institutional context and physical, policy, and suprapersonal factors appear to have comparable and mutually reinforcing influences on the type of social climate that emerges in a program.

Taken together, the four sets of predictors explain a substantial amount of the variance in residents' and staff members' perceptions of the treatment climate. In our sample of psychiatric and substance abuse programs, for example, the variance explained in residents' perceptions ranged from 45 percent for self-direction to 65 percent for self-understanding (mean = 57 percent); in staff members' perceptions it ranged from 40 percent for self-direction to 74 percent for practical orientation (mean = 58 percent) (Timko and Moos, 1996). More important, the relationships we found may help identify programs where interventions can contribute to a more supportive, resident-directed, and well-organized social climate than might otherwise develop.

Developing a Supportive Climate

The communal quality of psychiatric and substance abuse programs has both potential benefits and potential drawbacks. It offers the possibility of a supportive community to help individuals develop and sustain better personal relationships. By the same token, the enforced contacts in such settings may give rise to distress and conflict. An important goal for facility administrators is to establish a cohesive social climate in which conflict is low to moderate.

Managers and staff need to be aware of the interpersonal problems likely to arise among specific groups of residents. For example, programs drawing their residents population from less socially privileged or more mentally impaired groups are likely to develop less supportive treatment climates. Smaller programs and programs with staff members who function better together may be more able to counteract these tendencies with efforts aimed at reducing alienation and disharmony. A system in which designated staff teams ar responsible for specific groups of patients may also help to establish an involving and supportive social climate.

One way to enhance the quality of interpersonal engagement is to support the use of the program's public areas. An environment that is attractive, has features that foster social behavior and recreational activities, and offers adequate communal space encourages residents to use public areas and to be involved in positive interactions. The program can contribute to active involvement by providing a broad range of activities in these public areas and by offering opportunities for residents to meet for the purpose of jointly influencing program policies.

Along these lines, Bakos and his coworkers (1980) implemented an environmental management process by which residents and staff jointly planned changes to improve the physical design and social interaction in a treatment facility. Staff rearranged the dayroom furniture and constructed modular activity centers by introducing movable partitions and adding a kitchenette and snack area. The television set was placed in one corner of the dayroom where it would not be the central focus. New social activities were initiated. As expected, residents and staff spent more time in the dayroom. In addition, residents' activity levels increased and their behavior became more functional and adaptive. Residents who participated in the decisionmaking and change process showed the most improvement.

Another way to maintain residents' willingness to interact and to reduce conflict is to provide ample privacy. Opportunities to act without scrutiny by others and to withdraw from contact appear vital to sustaining supportive relationships and to reducing conflict. Residents also feel closer in settings where the physical environment allows staff to withdraw from direct contact with residents. Thus, in programs with little interpersonal warmth and much conflict, administrators can indirectly influence the social climate by increasing resident's' sense of control and privacy.

Enhancing Residents' Personal Development

A significant body of research supports the view that residents benefit from an emphasis on independence and from opportunities for personal development. Like the quality of relationships, the emphasis on resident's personal growth depends in part on predispositions that residents bring to the setting. Thus, for example, programs that draw their residents from the more socially advantaged and less cognitively impaired tend to place more emphasis on resident autonomy and on skills development and self-understanding. However, well-trained and experienced staff can encourage independence even when residents are impaired and in need of high levels of staff assistance.

The physical environment also can contribute to residents' self-direction. A physical environment that supports residents' engagement and activity by way of amenities and social-recreational aids can help communicate to residents that they are viewed as autonomous. The availability of adequate space for resident and staff functions also promotes the emphasis on independence.

Policies that provide residents formal input in decisionmaking and more choice in daily routines have a positive impact on residents' self-direction. Specifically, the development of a residents' council can have benefits in this area, even though residents emphasize the social and expressive functions of such councils more than their role in facility governance and policy formation. When staff members allow residents to make and implement important decisions, such councils are more likely to contribute to residents' sense of support and control. To promote independence and still maintain support and organization, staff need to help clients adhere to program schedules and participate in program activities.

Finally, to enhance an emphasis on independence, staff must be aware of its importance to residents and refrain from interfering with its exercise. Settings with greater staff resources tend to develop more emphasis on resident self-direction, as well as on self-understanding and the open expression of feelings. By identifying how particular staff characteristics are related to social climate, it may be possible to develop focused interventions. Thus, in-service training can deal with how staff may subtly undermine residents' efforts at independence. Program managers can help staff recognize how to encourage independent functioning and skills development rather than dependency.

Maintaining Organization

Administrators generally strive to have a well-organized program in which staff carry out their duties efficiently and in which residents are clear about rules and expectations. Achieving good organization is a greater challenge in large facilities and in those with residents who have fewer social or functional resources. However, administrators can avoid some of the potential negative effects of large size by intervening in specific processes in the program, for example, by taking steps to reduce the program's impersonal qualities. In addition, the presence of more women and older staff members contributes to organization, so that greater effort might be made to recruit and retain such staff.

Although physical features and policies are not strongly related to program structure, more amenities and more space for resident and staff functions are associated with better organization, as are clear policies. Managers may be able to enhance organization by reducing crowding and encouraging respect for residents' privacy needs, and by developing more formal mechanisms to communicate program policies to new residents and staff.

Improving the Social Climate

Our suggestions for improving social climate in treatment programs imply an active planning role for both residents and staff. To implement such changes effectively, we need better staff training and staff with more experience in psychological and behavioral areas. Winnett (1989) has emphasized the important role of mental health practitioners in promoting an environment oriented toward psychosocial rehabilitation. Consultants can work with psychologists and other similarly trained staff to assess and change specific aspects of the social climate and thereby promote optimum resident and staff functioning.

The process of identifying goals and planning change can benefit residents and staff members, who may often feel relatively powerless within a program. Although residents and staff may have somewhat different perspectives, their interests overlap; the majority of factors that contribute to residents' perceptions of support, self-direction, and good organization contribute similarly to staff members' perceptions. Having shown that physical features, policies and services, and aggregate resident and staff characteristics influence the treatment climate, we focus next on how the treatment climate affects residents' in-program and community adjustment.

9

In-Program Outcomes:
Satisfaction, Self-Confidence,
and Interpersonal Behavior

The research reported in this and the next two chapters examines the associations between the treatment environment and treatment outcome; that is, the connections between variables in panel III and panels IV and V in the conceptual model (figure 1.1). This chapter focuses on how hospital and community programs' treatment environments influence in-program outcomes, especially clients' satisfaction and self-confidence, interpersonal behavior, and dropout and turnover rates. Chapter 10 focuses on how hospital and community programs affect clients' readmission and adaptation in the community. Chapter 11 examines the evidence on client-program matching and extends the framework to consider how the health care workplace affects the treatment milieu and staff members' and clients' outcomes.

Although traditionally hospital and community programs have been examined separately, we consider them together for both practical and conceptual reasons. From a practical perspective, the number and diversity of community programs has grown rapidly in the last two decades and community programs now serve the full spectrum of clients with psychiatric and substance abuse disorders. Accordingly, many community programs offer a range of mental health and case management services that is comparable to the services offered in hospital programs. Moreover, rather than a dichotomy there is a continuum of care, including hospital-based hostels and partial hospitalization and day-care programs, and community-based halfway houses and intensive case management services.

From a conceptual point of view, the connections between treatment environment and outcome are likely to apply across program locations. The use of a common framework to examine the outcomes of diverse programs may help to broaden our knowledge about the common healing processes in hospital and community care. For the many clients seen in multiple hospital and community programs, it also makes it possible to examine the joint influence of the two loci of care.

Conceptual Rationale

As noted in chapter 1, one of the key assumptions underlying the development of different types of treatment programs is that the social environment influences clients' attitudes and behavior. This point is illustrated by Gunderson (1983), who focused on the diversification of milieu treatment and the growing evidence that such treatment can have quite powerful effects on clients' outcomes. There is also increased recognition that the emphasis on clients' interaction patterns and expression of affect must be balanced by an orientation toward skill development and program structure, especially for more disturbed individuals. In this respect, Paul and Menditto (1992) note that chronic mental patients do better in comprehensive social learning programs than in milieu-oriented or therapeutic community programs.

In terms of overall outcomes, we thought that programs that emphasize positive interpersonal relationships (involvement, support, and spontaneity), and high performance expectations with respect to self-direction, the development of work and social skills, and self-understanding would enhance clients' satisfaction and self-confidence and reduce their dropout and attrition rates. Because most clients need specific behavioral guidelines and structure, we expected that organization and clarity would also be associated with these outcomes. In addition, because most clients value their freedom and independence, we predicted that staff control would be linked to less satisfaction and self-confidence. We also expected that treatment environments would facilitate conceptually consonant coping styles; for example, more program emphasis on personal problem orientation should be associated with more client initiatives in the area of self-revelation.

Satisfaction and Self-Confidence

There is a considerable amount of information about clients' general reactions to treatment programs. In a review of early research in this area, Weinstein (1979) concluded that patients provide a rather more favorable picture of psychiatric programs than that drawn by critics of mental hospitals. Based on a more recent review and a study in a rural psychiatric facility, O'Mahoney and Ward (1995) conclude that long-term patients are modestly satisfied with their hospital life, perhaps because they have accommodated to it. Clients in group homes rate their quality of life as better than do clients in hospital or board-and-care facilities. Most important, clients' satisfaction and quality of life varies significantly among both hospital and community programs (Lehman, Slaughter, and Myers, 1991; MacDonald, Sibbald, and Hoare, 1988).

Hospital Programs

To focus on program-related correlates of patients' reactions, we examined the associations between the treatment environment in twenty-three hospital programs and patients' satisfaction and self-confidence. Patients were given the WAS and a set of items to assess: (1) their satisfaction with the program; (2) how much they liked the staff; (3) their anxiety; and (4) how much the program helped them increase their self-confidence (Moos, 1974; chapter 7).

Patients in involving, clear, and well-organized programs that emphasized autonomy and practical and personal problem orientation were more satisfied with treatment and the staff and thought they had a better chance to enhance their self-confidence (table 9.1). Less staff control was also associated with these three in-program outcome criteria. More program clarity was associated with less patient anxiety. (The support and spontaneity subscales were highly correlated with involvement in these programs and thus were dropped from the analyses.)

One potential explanation of these findings is that individual patients' response tendencies, such as a general inclination to answer questions either positively or negatively, mediate the associations between program characteristics and patients' reactions. To control for such influences, we randomly divided the patients in each of the twenty-

TABLE 9.1
Correlations between WAS Subscales and
Patients' Satisfaction and Morale

WAS Subscales	Patients' Satisfaction and Morale			
	General Satisfaction	Liking for Staff	Anxiety	Self-Confidence
Involvement	.77**	.52**	.06	.71**
Autonomy	.45*	.46*	-.13	.37+
Practical Orientation	.48**	.26	.12	.55**
Personal Problem Orientation	.75**	.65**	-.01	.65**
Anger and Aggression	.28	.39+	-.27	.21
Order and Organization	.70**	.33+	-.05	.47**
Program Clarity	.58**	.33+	-.42*	.27
Staff Control	-.62**	-.73**	.29	-.49*

Note. N=23 programs

+p <.10; **p <.05; ***p <.01

three programs into two groups. We obtained new means for the WAS subscales and patients' satisfaction and self-confidence for each of the two groups in each of the twenty-three programs. We then examined the program-level associations between the WAS subscale means of the first group of patients and the satisfaction and self-confidence scores of the second group, and those between the second group's WAS subscale means and the first group's outcomes.

The results were essentially identical to those shown in table 9.1. A total of nineteen of the twenty-one significant correlations between the WAS subscales and the indices of patients' in-program outcomes were essentially replicated in both pairs of the split sample. Only two correlations, those between organization and liking for staff and between program clarity and anxiety, were not replicated. These findings strengthen the idea that there are important connections between the treatment environment and patients' satisfaction and self-confidence. In addition, at the individual level of analysis, patients who report more emphasis on the relationship dimensions, on autonomy and practical orientation, and on organization and clarity, and less emphasis on staff control tend to be more satisfied with treatment (Bocker, 1989).

Community Programs

We have also examined this issue in community programs. Specifically, comparable to our work in hospital programs, we asked clients in thirteen community programs about their satisfaction with the program, how much they liked the staff, how anxious they felt, and how much they thought the program helped them enhance their self-confidence.

Clients in more supportive programs that emphasized self-direction and self-understanding tended to be more satisfied, to like the staff more, and to be more hopeful about treatment (Moos, 1974; chapter 12). Program organization and clarity were also associated with clients' satisfaction; in addition, clients in programs high on staff control tended to be less anxious. In a study of eighteen community programs, Davis (1985) found that residents in more supportive, self-directed, practically oriented, and well-organized programs were more satisfied. According to Fairchild and Wright (1984), adolescent clients who saw their programs as clearer, better organized, and less controlling were more satisfied. In general, these findings are comparable to those obtained in hospital programs.

Interpersonal Behavior and Adaptation

Through the treatment environment they create, psychiatric programs try to facilitate clients' coping and interpersonal behavior. To examine this issue, we developed measures of the main types of coping and helping behaviors clients show in psychiatric programs. We also focus here on indices of clients' communication and involvement, participation in treatment and use of program resources, and overall in-program adaptation.

Clients' Coping Behavior

We first developed a scale to assess four main aspects of patients' coping behavior in psychiatric programs: affiliation, self-revelation, aggression, and submission (Houts and Moos, 1969). The subscale items reflect specific initiatives that patients can take in treatment programs. For example, affiliation initiatives are inferred from items such as "I try to become friends with other patients in the program" and "If I am interested in a conversation I will join in and give my opinions." Self-revelation initiatives are inferred from the following items: "I try to share my personal problems with patients" and "I tell the staff about my feelings." Initiatives in the area of aggression are inferred from such items as: "I often criticize or joke about the staff" and "I sometimes argue for the fun of it." Finally, submission is inferred from such items as "I try to talk about things that the staff thinks are important" and "I do things that the staff ask me to do even if I don't like to."

We used these measures to focus on the relationships between the treatment environment and patients' initiatives in the twenty-three hospital programs in the study described earlier. Three main sets of findings emerged (table 9.2):

- When programs are high on involvement and personal problem orientation, patients rely more on initiatives in the areas of affiliation and self-revelation. When programs emphasize practical orientation and play down staff control, patients also rely more on these initiatives.
- When programs are involving, emphasize the open expression of anger, and are low on staff control patients rely more on aggression.
- When programs are involving, emphasize autonomy and the open expression of anger, and are low on staff control, patients are less submissive to the staff.

When we examined the associations between the WAS subscale means of the patients in one half of the split sample and the initiatives of the patients in the other half, the findings were essentially identical to those shown in table 9.2. All fifteen of the fifteen significant correlations in table 9.2 were statistically significant in either or both of the split sample analyses. Thus, the findings replicate when assessment of the treatment milieu and of patients' initiatives is based on different patient subsamples (Moos and Houts, 1970).

Overall, there is a quite specific pattern of relationships between the treatment environment and patients' coping responses. Highly involving programs promote patients' affiliative behavior; personal problem orientation facilitates patients' self-revelation; program focus on the expression of anger enhances patients' initiatives in this area. As staff control increases, patients' are more likely to be submissive; more-

TABLE 9.2
Correlations between WAS Subscales and Patients' Initiatives

WAS Subscales	Patients' Initiatives			
	Affiliation	Self-Revelation	Aggression	Submission
Involvement	.46*	.48**	.38+	-.37+
Autonomy	.06	.15	.26	-.41*
Practical Orientation	.53**	.43*	.23	.08
Personal Problem Orientation	.38+	.51**	.22	.23
Anger and Aggression	-.03	.38+	.67**	-.58**
Order and Organization	.14	.05	-.04	-.14
Program Clarity	-.02	-.13	.17	-.10
Staff Control	-.34+	-.32	-.43*	.57**

Note. N = 23 programs

+p <.10; *p <.05; **p <.01

over, patients' take fewer initiatives in the areas of affiliation, self-revelation, and the open expression of anger.

Clients' and Staff Members' Helping Behavior

The foregoing findings imply that treatment environments may influence patients in part because they affect how patients help each other and how staff help patients. Helping behaviors reflect the social matrix or mediating processes through which the treatment environment affects in-program and perhaps in-community outcomes. Accordingly, we focused on the associations between the treatment environment and patients' and staff members' helping styles.

Assessment of helping behavior. We administered a seventy-item Helping Scale to patients in nine programs. Patients answered each item twice on a seven-point scale in terms of the frequency with which (a) patients and (b) staff engaged in each of the helping behaviors (Sidman and Moos, 1973). In separate analyses on each of the two sets of seventy items, we identified three comparable factors that measured

(1) friendship behavior (for example, "One patient tries to help another" and "A staff member tries to be a patient's friend"); (2) enhancement of self-esteem (for example, "One patient treats another as a competent and responsible person" and "A staff member helps a patient accomplish something"); and (3) directive teaching (for example, "One patient helps another by getting him or her to follow a schedule" and "A staff member tries to teach a patient how to control his or her feelings better").

Treatment environment and helping behavior. We examined the program-level associations between the WAS subscale means and these helping styles. The findings for patients' helping behavior show that:

- patients in supportive and well-organized programs that emphasize the development of work and social skills report more helping behavior in the areas of friendship and enhancement of self-esteem; and
- when programs play down autonomy and are high on staff control, patients report more directive teaching.

The results for staff helping behaviors show that:

- patients in supportive and well-organized programs report that staff are more likely to help them by enhancing their self-esteem; and
- patients in supportive and well-organized programs that also place more emphasis on the development of work and social skills and less on the open expression of anger report that staff engage in more friendship behavior and directive teaching.

The results described earlier point to relationships between specific aspects of treatment environments and patients' satisfaction and coping behavior. This study generalizes the findings to patients' and staff members' helping styles. Most broadly, supportive and well-organized programs promote patients' and staff members' praising patients and enhancing their self-confidence. An emphasis on patients' work and social skills also fosters reliance on these helping behaviors. Highly structured programs increase patients' reliance on helping each other by directive teaching. In all likelihood, patients' and staff members' helping behavior mediates the connections between specific aspects of the treatment environment and other in-program outcomes, such as satisfaction and self-confidence.

Communication and Involvement

According to Alden (1978b), there is some connection between treatment environments, outside observers' ratings of patient-staff interaction, and staff members' ratings of changes in patients' interpersonal behavior. Programs that were more supportive, expressive, and self-directed had more social interaction among patients and between patients and staff. These programs were also higher on practical and personal problem orientation. Program with more social interaction contributed to improvement in patients' activity levels, self-care, and depression.

There were also some connections between the treatment environment and changes in patients' behavior over a three-month interval. In supportive programs that emphasized self-understanding and the open expression of anger, patients communicated more but also became more belligerent. Programs that were higher on self-understanding and expressiveness contributed to improvements in patients' self-care abilities. In contrast, patients in programs high on staff control became less communicative and more seclusive. Thus, although staff control contributes to smooth program operations, it may not facilitate patients' social functioning.

Aggressive behavior. There is strong evidence that contextual factors, such as overcrowded programs that lack structured activities and organization, are associated with patients' aggressive behavior (Finnema, Dassen, and Halfens, 1994; Flannery, Hansen, and Penk, 1994). To examine the program-level associations between the treatment climate and patients' aggressive behavior, we obtained information about the number of patients who engaged in aggressive behavior in a thirty-day interval in 143 hospital programs (Moos, 1974; chapter 6). When programs had less emphasis on autonomy, self-understanding, and the open expression of angry feelings, patients showed more aggressive behavior (see also Moos, 1972c). According to Lanza et al. (1994), a lack of autonomy and high staff control were modestly associated with more patient assaults.

In the study of twenty-three programs described earlier, we tabulated the number of behavior incidents in each program over a four-month interval and examined the associations between the treatment environment and such incidents. When programs lacked involvement and spontaneity and were low on practical and personal problem orientation, patients engaged in more aggressive behavior; this was also true in programs that staff saw as less clear and well-organized. These findings reflect the importance of supportive and well-structured programs, as well as the difficulty in organizing such programs for more disturbed patients.

Engagement in group treatment. Some aspects of the treatment environment are associated with participation and specific patterns of interaction in group meetings. Thus, Friis (1986b) developed an interaction score that reflected in part the amount of time patients spent each week in patient-staff group meetings. When programs were higher on involvement, autonomy, and self-understanding and lower on staff control patients spent more time in group meetings.

The process and proximal outcome of group therapy in a program may also mediate part of the association between the treatment environment and patients' in-program outcomes. In Kahn, Storke, and Schaeffer's (1992) study, patients and staff attending a weekly community meeting described the treatment environment; patients and staff attending focus and discussion groups rated the group process. High support and spontaneity in the treatment program predicted patients' engagement in the groups, specifically their cohesion, self-disclosure, and willingness to confront other patients. A lack of practical orientation and clarity in the program predicted conforming and superficial behavior in the groups. Finally, high anger and lack of organization in the program were associated with group conflict. Thus, there were some conceptually meaningful relationships between the overall treatment environment and patients' behavior in the groups.

Participation in activities and use of services. We have examined these issues in program-level analyses of a national sample of 262 residential facilities for older adults (Moos and Lemke, 1994; chapter 8). Even after controlling for residents' social resources and functional abilities, specific aspects of social climate were predictably associated with residents' in-program adaptation. Specifically, residents in more cohesive and independence-oriented facilities were more likely to be involved in activities in the community and relied less on facility services; outside observers also saw them as better adjusted. Residents in better organized facilities that were low on conflict and independence were more likely to participate in planned activities in the facility. In facilities with a high level of resident influence, residents were less likely to use the available health services and were rated as better adjusted.

Overall In-Program Adaptation

Accurate expectations about a treatment program should help newly admitted clients adapt better to it. Thus, patients on admission units who expected the staff to be helpful saw the program as more open, tolerant, and oriented to personal problems over time (Lieberman et al., 1992). We focused on this issue in four community programs to find out whether new clients whose expectations matched those of clients already in the program would make better use of the program. New clients who have more realistic expectations about a program may develop better relationships with staff, participate more actively in the program, and be more likely to follow the staff's treatment recommendations.

We used the COPES Form E (Expectations) to measure prospective clients' expectations of the community program to which they were referred. The COPES Form E is composed of 100 items and ten subscales that are parallel to Form R (Moos, 1996a). The four programs were a client-run program in a VA medical center, two day-care centers, and a day hospital. Staff members rated new clients as well adjusted (that is, as attending regularly, participating well, and making reasonably good use of the program) or as poorly adjusted. A total of forty-seven patients were rated as well-adjusted and twenty-six as poorly adjusted. Clients already in the four programs reported on the treatment environment, as did the new clients who remained in their program for one to two months.

We first compared successful and unsuccessful clients' initial expectations. Clients who later adapted well in the program had more realistic expectations than did clients who later adapted poorly. More specifically, compared with the actual program, the unsuccessful clients expected that their program would be much more supportive and expressive, much clearer, and have much more emphasis on self-direction, self-understanding, and the development of work and social skills (Otto and Moos, 1974).

The successful clients in all four programs tended to change their perceptions of the program between the time they entered it and one or two months later. After these changes occurred, new clients' perceptions matched those of existing clients more closely. Thus, when clients' initial expectations are moderately discrepant from actual program characteristics, these perceptions tend to change and become more accurate with experience in the program.

In general, patients tend to improve substantially between admission and discharge and to be moderately or highly satisfied with treatment (Coyne et al., 1990). Patients who obtain clear information and participate in planning their treatment improve more; satisfaction with care is also associated with in-program improvement (Hansson, 1989; Hansson and Berglund, 1987). One important issue for further research is to find out whether clients' satisfaction with treatment predicts their longer-term outcomes.

Another important issue is to examine the extent to which clients and staff attribute the therapeutic value of treatment to different factors. Consistent with our findings, Goldstein et al. (1988) noted that chronically mentally ill day hospital clients who portrayed their program as supportive and clear were more likely to see the program as helpful. Contrary to our findings and to staff members' reports, however, clients who saw less emphasis on personal problem orientation rated the program as more helpful. These findings may reflect the detrimental influence of a strong emphasis on self-disclosure on severely mentally ill clients. More broadly, to plan and implement effective programs, we need more information on clients' reactions to varied treatment programs and components.

Dropout and Attrition Rates

Dropout rates are seldom used as proximal indicators of treatment outcome. However, program dropout rates are substantial: An average of 20 percent to 30 percent of the patients in many of the programs we studied dropped out of treatment. Moreover, programs with high dropout rates clearly are ineffective with a certain proportion of patients; high program dropout rates are associated with higher casemix-adjusted readmission rates (Peterson et al., 1994; Swindle et al., 1995). Accordingly, more information is needed about the program characteristics that give rise to high dropout rates. As we saw earlier (chapter 3), such information can motivate staff to improve the treatment environment and thus reduce dropout rates (Verinis, 1983).

Research in this area has focused on program-level associations between the treatment environment and patients' dropout rates, as well as on individual-level associations between patients' perceptions of a program and the likelihood that they will drop out of the program.

Program Environment and Dropout Rate

In an initial project, we tried to identify characteristics of treatment environments that were consistently associated with program dropout rates. We focused on two groups of programs that differed in their average size. One set of eight programs was relatively small, averaging twenty-six patients. The staffing ratios in these programs were similar, although the smaller programs had slightly richer staffing. The patients in these VA programs were all men; their average age was about forty years; more than 80 percent were single, widowed, or divorced; more than 65 percent were diagnosed schizophrenic; the vast majority had been hospitalized previously, most more than once. The only variable that significantly differentiated among the programs was patients' median length of stay in the hospital, indicating that the programs were closely comparable.

The second set of seven programs was relatively large, varying from seventy-three to 129 patients. The patient-staff ratio varied from 3.7 to 5.6 patients for each staff member. Patients were randomly assigned to these programs; if readmission became necessary, patients were returned to the program from which they had been discharged. Accordingly, patients' background characteristics were closely comparable across programs. For example, 62 percent of all discharged patients were diagnosed schizophrenic; this varied from 57 percent to 72 percent across programs. The percentage of discharged patients who were married averaged 38 percent and varied from 30 percent to 43 percent (Moos and Schwartz, 1972).

We focused on program differences in the percentage of patients who left the hospital without permission or against medical advice during a six-month interval in the small programs and a three-month interval in the large programs. The programs differed significantly in dropout rates. The dropout rate varied from 4 percent to 45 percent among the small programs and from 32 percent to 79 percent among the large programs. Patients and staff members in each program completed the WAS. We then examined the associations between the percentage of patients or staff members in each program who answered true to each WAS item and the program dropout rate (Moos, 1974, chapter 8; Moos, Shelton, and Petty, 1973).

Programs with high dropout rates. A substantial number of WAS items were moderately to highly correlated with program dropout rates.

Specifically, patients' perceptions on thirty items in the small programs and on twenty-nine items in the large programs correlated .40 or higher with dropout rates. This was also true of staff members' perceptions on forty-three items in the small programs and forty-eight items in the large programs. The next step was to identify a combination of WAS items that was consistently associated with the dropout rate. We then constructed a scale composed of fifteen WAS items that was highly correlated with the dropout rate in both sets of programs.

The rank-order correlations between patients' and staff members' scores on the fifteen-item dropout scale and the dropout rate were .90 and .97, respectively, in the eight small programs and .82 and .86, respectively, in the seven large programs. Patients and staff agreed that the fifteen items were characteristic of programs with high dropout rates; rank-order correlations over programs between patients' and staff members' dropout scale scores were .93 for the eight small programs and .61 for the seven large programs.

Table 9.3 shows the fifteen items on the dropout scale grouped by content area. The scoring direction is given for each item. Patients and staff see programs with high dropout rates as uninvolved and nonsupportive, low on autonomy, and disorganized and unclear. Programs with high dropout rates have few social activities and little emphasis on involving patients in the program or carefully planning patients' activities. Staff are not interested in learning about patients' feelings and do not go out of their way to help patients. Staff also discourage criticism from patients and are unwilling to act on patients' suggestions. Patients often complain or criticize the staff, perhaps because the program is poorly organized and patients have no regular daily schedule.

Bell (1985) obtained comparable findings in three Second Genesis programs for clients with drug abuse problems. Two of the programs had well-implemented, structured therapeutic communities; the third program was much less supportive and less oriented toward clients' personal growth. The client dropout rate was much higher in the poorly implemented than in the two well-implemented programs (26 percent versus an average of 14 percent). Similarly, Keso and Salaspuro (1990) found a much lower dropout rate in a Hazelden-type program than in a comparison program (8 percent versus 26 percent); the Hazelden-type program was much more supportive and well organized and more oriented toward self-understanding.

TABLE 9.3
Dropout Scale Items and Scoring Key

WAS Item Number and Scale	Scored Direction	Item
51. Involvement	False	Patients are quite busy all the time.
61. Involvement	True	The program has very few social activities.
96. Unscored	True	It is hard to get a group together for card games or other activities.
92. Support	False	Staff go out of their way to help patients.
4. Autonomy	False	The staff act on patients' suggestions.
94. Autonomy	True	The staff discourage criticism.
66. Personal Problem	False	Staff are mainly interested in learning about patients' feelings.
7. Anger	True	Patients often gripe.
17. Anger	True	Patients often criticize or joke about the staff.
8. Order	False	Patients' activities are carefully planned.
18. Order	False	This is a very well-organized program.
48. Order	False	Most patients follow a regular schedule each day.
58. Order	True	Many patients look messy.
68. Order	True	Things are sometimes very disorganized around here.
59. Clarity	False	In this program, everyone knows who is in charge.

Dropout rates among youth. Program characteristics associated with dropout among youth appear to be similar to those associated with dropout among adults. In this vein, Friedman and Glickman (1987) focused on the case failure rate (the proportion of clients who left before completing treatment or who were incarcerated or discharged for noncompliance with program rules) in twenty-two residential programs for youth. Even after controlling for program differences in clients' demographic characteristics, programs that emphasized practical assistance in solving clients' real-life problems, self-understanding, and expressive personal relationships had lower client failure rates.

In another study, an adapted version of the COPES was used to describe group home treatment environments. Compared with residents from nonsupportive and authoritarian homes, residents from supportive and participatory homes felt more positively about their experience in the home and were less likely to run away from it and become recidivists (Patton, 1977).

Dropout rate as a proximal index of treatment outcome. Overall, the findings show that clients are more likely to drop out of programs that are not well-implemented. However, clients who are not ready to participate fully in treatment may find it hard to adapt to programs that have an active and directed treatment orientation. Such programs may have an elevated dropout rate. Accordingly, Leda, Rosenheck, and Fontana (1991) found that residential programs for homeless veterans that were higher on a therapeutic activity index (more emphasis on relationship and personal growth dimensions) had a larger proportion of clients who were discharged involuntarily.

Similarly, in a comparison of three therapeutic community programs for substance abuse patients, Bale and his colleagues (1984) found a high attrition rate in the two programs that demanded new members' immediate involvement and participation. The highest attrition was in the program that also had a lack of clarity, organization, and staff control. To reduce attrition in highly demanding, directed treatment programs, staff may need to establish supportive relationships with clients and allow them to engage in treatment somewhat gradually.

Clients' Perceptions and Attrition

Subsequent studies in this area have identified associations between individual clients' perceptions of a treatment program and the likelihood that the client will drop out of the program. In this respect, a client's perception of the treatment milieu may reflect the working alliance between the client and treatment personnel and may encourage or discourage continuation in the program and in treatment.

Clients' perceptions, dropout, and aftercare. We analyzed the relationship between individual clients' perceptions of the social climate and their likelihood of dropping out of a Salvation Army substance abuse program. Clients who dropped out of the program did not differ from the rest of the clients in personal resources on admission, but they appraised the treatment milieu more negatively than did their counterparts who remained in the program. Specifically, the dropouts saw the program as less involving, supportive, clear, and well organized (Moos, Mehren, and Moos, 1978).

According to Vaglum et al. (1990), clients who see their program as less supportive and well organized and less oriented toward the development of work and social skills, are more likely to drop out or leave the program against medical advice. Clients' reports of low spontaneity and staff control have also been associated with dropout in admissions programs (Tessier, 1990). In contrast, clients who see their program as encouraging self-direction, self-understanding, and the open expression of anger may be more likely to participate in outpatient aftercare groups led by program staff members (Pratt et al., 1977). Clients who are better integrated into a treatment program are more likely to continue in outpatient treatment, which is associated with better treatment outcome (Peterson et al., 1994; Swindle et al., 1995).

Clients' perceptions of the program may also be associated with the type of discharge. Specifically, clients in a drug treatment program who thought that the open expression of anger was less acceptable were more likely to be discharged due to disciplinary problems than to be regular dropouts (Harris, Linn, and Pratt, 1980). Compared with clients who openly drop out, clients who are discharged because of their problem behavior may be less willing to accept direct responsibility for their decision to leave the program. That is, clients who report that the expression of aggression is negatively sanctioned may engage in problem behavior in order to be dismissed from the program.

Because of their very short duration and clients' greater needs for treatment, however, these findings may not hold in detoxification (detox) programs. In fact, in a standard heroin detox program and in an experimental outpatient detox clinic, Hall and her colleagues (1979) found that clients' perceptions of the treatment milieu were unrelated to whether they dropped out or completed treatment.

Clients' demographic characteristics as moderators. Sociodemographic factors such as age, race, and gender may moderate the association between clients' perceptions of the treatment program and attrition. Linn (1978) linked older (over fifty-five) and younger (under fifty) alcoholic clients' perceptions of the treatment climate in a therapeutic community program to their attrition rates. Older clients who reported a lack of involvement, spontaneity, and autonomy were more likely to leave the program; in contrast, younger clients who reported more autonomy were more likely to drop out. Linn (1978) speculated that it is especially important for older clients to feel included in treatment and to be encouraged to be self-sufficient and independent; in addition, younger clients may need more structure to encourage them to remain in treatment.

A more therapeutic milieu may be especially salient for African-American drug abuse clients, perhaps because they constitute a minority group in many treatment programs. Linn and her colleagues (1979) examined the connection between race and attrition among men in a therapeutic community program. African-American clients who saw the program as more spontaneous, and oriented more toward independence, the development of work and social skills, and self-understanding were more likely to remain in treatment. These findings did not hold for Caucasian clients, who constituted the majority of the clients in the program.

In another study of a therapeutic community program, Doherty (1976) found that clients who acted in accord with the program's normative expectations (such as by being more self-confident, being more likely to help other patients, and engaging in more self-disclosure) were discharged more quickly. Among men, those who saw the program as better organized tended to remain in the program longer, perhaps because they thought that a structured setting would benefit them. Consistent with the idea that women may find it hard to adapt to a strong demand for self-disclosure in a mixed-gender treatment setting, women who reported more emphasis on personal problem orientation tended to leave the program sooner.

Turnover Rates

The program turnover or discharge rate is a measure of a program's efficiency in returning hospitalized clients to a more normative residential facility or to an independent placement in the community. The discharge rate is an important criterion of program functioning; however, it is determined in part by aspects of the community environment, such as the existence of supportive services and the clients' family and work settings.

In a study of nineteen programs in five VA medical centers, Ellsworth and his coworkers (1971) found that, in programs with high turnover rates, nursing staff reported that they received less praise for their work and that the professional staff were less well motivated. Programs with high turnover rates tended not to promote client autonomy. These findings imply that high turnover units are run by professional staff who do not take the time to involve clients or staff in responsible roles and instead focus primarily on admitting and discharging clients.

Identifying Programs with High Discharge Rates

We used the data from the two sets of VA programs described earlier to examine the associations between the treatment environment and program discharge rates. We focused on patients who were discharged during a six-month interval in the eight small programs and a three-month interval in the seven large programs. The discharge rate was the number of patients who were discharged from each program divided by the number who were admitted to the program in the three-month or six-month interval. Patients who left a program without permission or were discharged against medical advice were not included.

The programs in both studies differed significantly in discharge rates. Specifically, the discharge rate varied from 38 percent to 159 percent among the eight small programs, and from 76 percent to 167 percent among the seven large programs. In a procedure that was comparable to the one we used to develop the dropout scale, we identified a set of fourteen WAS items that, according to both patients' and staff members' perceptions, was consistently associated with the discharge rate in both sets of programs.

The rank-order correlations between patients' and staff members' scores on the fourteen-item discharge scale and the discharge rate were .83 and .74, respectively, in the eight small programs, and .82 for both groups in the seven large programs. The discharge scale scores were not significantly associated with program dropout rates, indicating that aspects of the treatment milieu that contribute to high turnover rates are independent of those that contribute to high dropout rates. Patients' and staff members' discharge scale scores correlated .86 for the eight small programs and .79 for the seven large programs, indicating substantial agreement about the characteristics of high discharge rate programs.

The Treatment Milieu in High Discharge Rate Programs

Of the fourteen items on the discharge scale (see table 9.4), five are from the practical orientation subscale. Programs with high discharge rates strongly emphasize the development of patients' work and social skills and, as expected, making concrete plans for patients' discharge. High discharge rate programs also are quite structured; for example, patients must follow the schedule arranged for them.

High discharge rate programs are moderately supportive, but they do not encourage patients to become involved with the program or to express their feelings openly. Staff are interested in the patients and tell them when they are making progress, and the patients are proud of the program. However, patients are careful about what they say to the doctors, they rarely argue, and they tend to keep their disagreements to themselves. In this context, when staff ask patients personal questions it probably is more to gather information than to enhance self-disclosure. Overall, the primary focus in high discharge rate programs is on practical decisionmaking and information gathering in a somewhat unexpressive context.

These findings are consistent with Ellsworth and his colleagues (1971), who noted that programs with high discharge rates tended to play down patients' autonomy and that staff perceived them somewhat negatively. Similarly, compared with a longer-term treatment program, Squire (1994) noted that three short-term admission units were lower on involvement, autonomy, practical orientation, and the open expression of anger. In Friis' (1986b) study of thirty-five short-term programs, however, an emphasis on personal problem orientation was associated with more patient turnover, perhaps because a high proportion of the patients were acutely disturbed and could not adapt to the expectations for self-disclosure.

Treatment Environments and In-Program Outcomes

We have identified some general relationships between aspects of the treatment environment and clients' in-program outcomes. Most broadly, clients in supportive programs that emphasize self-direction, the development of work and social skills, and self-understanding tend to be more satisfied with treatment and to report that treatment enhances their self-confidence. Clients in well-organized and clear pro-

TABLE 9.4
Discharge Scale Items and Scoring Key

WAS Item Number and Scale	Scored Direction	Item
21. Involvement	True	The patients are proud of this program.
41. Involvement	True	Very few patients ever volunteer around here.
12. Support	False	The staff know what the patients want.
13. Spontaneity	False	Patients say anything they want to the doctors.
53. Spontaneity	True	When patients disagree with each other, they keep it to themselves.
5. Practical	True	New treatment approaches are often tried in this program.
25. Practical	True	Patients are strongly encouraged to plan for the future.
45. Practical	False	There is very little emphasis on making plans for leaving this program.
55. Practical	True	This program emphasizes training for new kinds of jobs.
95. Practical	True	Patients must make specific plans before leaving the program.
56. Personal Problem	False	The staff rarely ask patients personal questions.
27. Anger	True	Patients in this program rarely argue.
99. Clarity	True	Staff tells patients when they are getting better.
60. Control	True	Once a schedule is arranged for a patient, the patient must follow it.

grams that play down staff control also do better on these in-program outcomes. In general, these findings apply in both hospital and community programs.

The associations between the treatment environment and clients' coping behavior are more focused. Specific aspects of the program are linked to clients' initiatives in consonant areas. Program involvement promotes clients' affiliation; personal problem orientation facilitates clients' self-revelation; a focus on anger enhances clients' expression of anger. High staff control makes it more likely that clients will passively follow staff directives; it is also associated with low client morale and self-confidence, less affiliation and open discussion of personal problems, and less liking for staff members.

Supportive and well-organized programs that emphasize the development of work and social skills also facilitate clients' positive interpersonal behavior, especially being friendly to other clients and trying to enhance their self-esteem. Moreover, clients in such programs are less likely to engage in overt aggressive behavior; more emphasis on autonomy and self-understanding is also associated with less aggressive behavior.

These aspects of the treatment environment are also linked to clients' dropout rates and engagement in treatment. Programs that lack focus on the relationship and system maintenance areas have high dropout rates; clients who report less focus on these areas are more likely to leave treatment prematurely. Engagement in treatment seems to be more dependent on an emphasis on clients' personal growth, especially autonomy and self-understanding. Overall, these findings show that a supportive, well-organized treatment environment that is somewhat self-directed and sets moderate to strong performance expectations contributes to clients' better in-program outcomes. Next we focus on whether such treatment environments enhance clients' adjustment in the community.

10

Adaptation in the Community

We turn now to examine the connections between the treatment environment and clients' adaptation in the community. We focus specifically on clients' community tenure, symptom reduction and psychosocial functioning, and social integration and community living skills. These are distal program outcomes that reflect in part effective discharge planning and how well the program has prepared clients for independent or assisted living in the community. In this chapter, we examine the direct connections between specific aspects of the treatment climate and clients' community outcomes; that is, between variables in panels III and V of the conceptual framework (see figure 1.1). In chapter 11 we focus on how clients' personal characteristics (panel II in the model), especially the severity of their mental impairment, influence the associations between program characteristics and outcomes.

From a broader perspective, a treatment program is only one among many sets of factors that influence clients' community adjustment. Specific aspects of clients' life contexts, especially stressful life circumstances and the characteristics of family and work settings, and clients' cognitive and behavioral coping skills, shape long-term post-treatment functioning (Moos, Finney, and Cronkite, 1990). Nevertheless, because treatment programs change individuals in ways that affect their adjustment after discharge, more information is needed about the specific links between program processes and outcomes.

In light of the fact that psychiatric patients have been treated in hospital and community residential programs for more than 150 years, it is surprising that relatively little is known about the connections between specific aspects of treatment environments and patients' adaptation in the community. A host of studies have shown that, on average, psychiatric and substance abuse patients experience substantial improvement between admission to inpatient treatment and six- to twelve-month follow-ups (e.g. Blotcky, Dimperio, and Gossett, 1984; Deering et al., 1991; Polich, Armor, and Braiker, 1981); however, these studies obtained little or no systematic information about program treatment environments. Long-term follow-ups of intensively treated patients also show improvement for some groups of patients, but again such improvement has not been linked to the treatment climate (McGlashan, 1984, 1986).

In one relevant study, Ellsworth and his coworkers (1971) identified some characteristics of programs with low readmission rates. These programs had motivated professional staff and active participant roles for both nursing staff and patients. Nursing staff saw themselves as involved in treatment planning and being praised for their work. Accordingly, the program characteristics associated with high discharge rates (see chapter 9) may be somewhat different from those related to the likelihood that discharged patients will remain in the community.

Community Tenure Rates

One measure of program success is the extent to which patients remain in the community; that is, are not readmitted for additional inpatient psychiatric or substance abuse care. Readmission following inpatient care is a key measure of services utilization and may be a valuable indicator of quality of care. Readmission is associated with poor posttreatment functioning, is costly, and, by targeting resources for a small group of recurrent patients, may delay treatment for other individuals. Program readmission or community tenure rates are easily monitored through secondary data sources; accordingly, it is quite inexpensive to obtain this information.

To address this issue, we relied on the data from the two sets of VA programs described earlier (chapter 9). We focused on patients who were discharged to an independent placement in the community and defined a program's community tenure rate as the percentage of discharged patients who were still in the community after six months in the eight small programs and three months in the seven large programs. Patients who left their program without permission or were discharged against medical advice were not included. In addition, we did not obtain information about patients' readmissions to non-VA hospitals.

The community tenure rate varied from 11 percent to 76 percent in the eight small programs and from 78 percent to 89 percent in the seven large programs. Following the logic we used to develop the dropout and discharge rate scales (chapter 9), we identified a set of twelve WAS items that were related to the community tenure rate in both large and small programs.

The Treatment Climate in High Community Tenure Rate Programs

Patients' and staff members' scores on the twelve-item community tenure scale were closely associated with the community tenure criterion. The correlations were .82 for patients and .97 for staff in the eight small programs and .71 for patients and .79 for staff in the seven large programs. There was a high level of agreement between patients' and staff members' scores on the community tenure scale—.90 for the eight small programs and .86 for the seven large programs. Neither patients' nor staff members' perceptions were associated with program dropout or discharge rates, except for a significant correlation between patients' perceptions and dropout in the eight small programs. Thus, the community tenure scale basically is uniquely related to community tenure.

The twelve items in the community tenure scale (table 10.1) describe a structured program that emphasizes patients' autonomy and the development of their work and social skills. Patients are encouraged to be independent and the staff treat them with respect, but patients are transferred out of the program if they do not obey the rules. These programs also value self-understanding and the open expression of feelings, especially anger.

Broadly speaking, programs that keep patients out of the hospital function similarly to high discharge rate programs in several areas; that is, they emphasize practical orientation in a relatively structured program context. However, high community tenure programs encourage self-understanding and the open expression of feelings, whereas high discharge rate programs do not.

To examine the applicability of these findings in a high-risk diagnostic group, we focused specifically on unmarried schizophrenic patients' community tenure. These patients typically are acutely dis-

TABLE 10.1
Community Tenure Scale Items and Scoring Key

WAS Item Number and Scale	Scored Direction	Item
83. Spontaneity	True	Patients are strongly encouraged to show their feelings.
34. Autonomy	True	Patients here are encouraged to be independent
35. Practical	False	There is very little emphasis on what patients will be doing after they leave.
75. Practical	True	Patients are encouraged to learn new ways of doing things.
36. Personal Problem	True	Patients are expected to share their personal problems with each other.
37. Anger	True	Staff sometimes argue openly with each other.
67. Anger	False	Staff here never start arguments.
77. Anger	True	In this program, staff think it is a healthy thing to argue.
78. Order	True	The staff set an example for neatness and orderliness.
88. Order	True	Patients are rarely kept waiting when they have appointments with staff.
80. Control	True	Patients will be transferred from this program is they do not obey the rules.
97. Unscored	False	A lot of patients just seem to be passing time here.

turbed and may respond more positively to program structure. Moreover, they have the fewest community ties and may be most reactive to the treatment environment. Schizophrenic patients who were treated in highly structured programs, as reflected by an emphasis on practical orientation and staff control, remained in the community for a longer interval after discharge (Moos and Schwartz, 1972).

Due to the small number of programs involved in this project, we were not able to control for program differences in patient casemix. However, we performed some additional analyses to examine the relationship between patients' demographic and diagnostic characteristics and prior treatment history and the community tenure rate. In essence, there were no significant program-level associations between the proportion of married patients, the proportion of schizophrenic patients, and the median length of patients' prior hospital stay, and either the community tenure scale or community tenure itself. These results suggest that the association between the community tenure scale and community tenure was not mediated by patients' prognostic characteristics. Nevertheless, the findings need to be replicated using more rigorous methods to control for program differences in patient-related prognostic factors.

Profiles of High and Low Community Tenure Rate Programs

To illustrate these findings, figure 10.1 shows staff members' perceptions of the program with the highest (HiCT) and the lowest (LoCT) community tenure rate. Staff in the HiCT program described an active, treatment-oriented milieu that was well above average in all three relationship and all four personal growth areas. Staff also reported that the program was clear and well organized but quite low on staff control.

The LoCT program's treatment milieu was quite different. Staff reported only moderate involvement and support and relatively little emphasis on the development of work and social skills or on self-understanding. Even though the LoCT program had some emphasis on autonomy, it was not well organized and staff exerted little effort to prepare patients for independent life in the community or to help them confront their personal problems. In this context, the elevated focus on expressiveness and anger is likely to reflect an uncontrolled venting of feelings rather than a constructive exploration of patients' problems.

FIGURE 10.1
WAS Form R Profiles for Staff on High and
Low Community Tenure Units

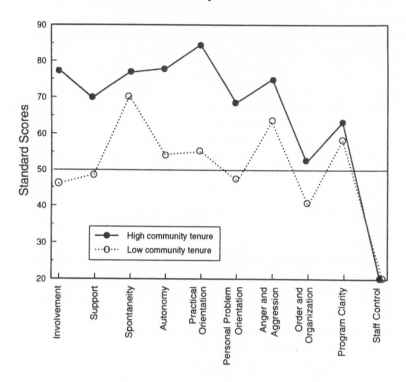

Compared with patients in the LoCT program, patients in the HiCT program reported more emphasis on autonomy and practical and personal problem orientation (not shown). Patients in the two programs appraised the relationship and system maintenance dimensions similarly, except for more staff control in the LoCT program. Thus, according to both patients and staff, the highest community tenure rate program had much more emphasis on patients' personal development.

Treatment Orientation and Community Tenure

These findings imply that a program's treatment goals, such as the emphasis on practical and personal problem orientation, have an especially important influence on clients' community tenure. Accordingly, we developed The Drug and Alcohol Program Treatment Inventory (DAPTI) to measure eight main treatment orientations characteristic of psychiatric and substance abuse programs (Swindle, et al., 1995). These orientations include cognitive behavioral, therapeutic community, family systems, and medical, as well as vocational rehabilitation and psychodynamic. To assess each orientation, we focus on general treatment goals, such as clients' accepting more responsibility for their decisions and actions, and on the specific treatment activities staff employ to help clients achieve these goals, such as teaching clients ways to manage their anger.

We used the DAPTI to characterize VA substance abuse programs and to examine the influence of program treatment orientations on readmission rates. In a project that focused on 88 programs, we found that the associations between treatment orientations and casemix-adjusted readmission rates varied by clients' age group (Moos, Mertens, and Brennan, 1995).

- Among younger clients (eighteen to thirty-four years of age), an emphasis on the development of social skills, vocational rehabilitation, personal responsibility as reflected by a therapeutic community orientation, and more family involvement in treatment was associated with lower readmission rates.
- Among middle-aged clients (thirty-five to fifty-four years of age), an emphasis on vocational rehabilitation was the main treatment orientation associated with lower readmission rates. Family involvement in treatment also predicted better outcomes.
- Among late middle-aged and older clients (fifty-five years of age or older), none of the program orientations were associated with readmission. In contrast, more structured program policies, more flexible rules about discharge, and less intensive treatment predicted lower readmission rates.

Consistent with our results on treatment climate, an emphasis on social and vocational skills was associated with lower readmission rates, but only among younger clients. Thus, substance abuse programs' treatment goals may have a stronger influence on younger than on older clients. Earlier, we saw that programs with more older clients had less involving treatment climates that were less oriented toward clients' autonomy, skills development, and self-understanding (chapter 8). These findings may help to explain why program goals are less likely to have an impact on older clients' outcomes.

Enhancing Community Tenure

Broadly speaking, these findings are consistent with those of other studies of programs that are successful in keeping clients out of hospital. For example, programs that emphasize stress management training and are more likely to involve family members and friends in assessment and treatment planning tend to have lower casemix-adjusted readmission rates (Peterson et al., 1994). Such programs may tailor treatment plans more effectively to enhance clients' relapse-prevention skills and address relationship issues between clients and important members of their social network. In this respect, Spencer et al. (1988) found that a psychoeducationally oriented inpatient family intervention was associated with improved individual and family functioning at follow-up, particularly among women with affective disorder or schizophrenia.

Among clients who have both substance abuse and psychiatric disorders, programs that are more tolerant of problem behavior have lower casemix-adjusted readmission rates (Swindle, et al., 1995). Clients who have multiple behavioral and psychological problems may find it hard to adapt in programs with harsh and controlling rules. Dually diagnosed clients in programs with more stringent policies may feel that staff are more likely to confront them about rules that seem arbitrary and not clearly related to their treatment goals. Similarly, when family members and friends were tolerant of their problem behavior, chronically mentally ill individuals were more satisfied with their community living circumstances (Sommers, 1987).

In essence, programs that are successful in keeping clients out of the hospital emphasize independence, work and social skills, self-understanding, and the open expression of anger; they are well-organized and have a moderate level of staff control. Clients in these programs also tend to have better in-program outcomes. The findings presented earlier (chapter 9) imply that clients in high community tenure programs generally are satisfied, think they can enhance their self-confidence in the program, and report that other clients and staff help them to develop friendships and self-confidence. These better in-program outcomes may foreshadow and contribute to better community outcomes.

Symptom Reduction and Psychosocial Functioning

Therapeutic Community Programs

More than forty years ago, therapeutic communities (TCs) became an important treatment modality for individuals with substance abuse disorders (Jones, 1953; Kennard, 1983). These TCs typically emphasize peer support, high performance expectations, and substantial structure as reflected by both client-controlled sanctions and strict staff-initiated rules and regulations. In practice, of course, TCs vary considerably in their underlying treatment philosophy and in their actual treatment environment.

Bale and his colleagues (1984) examined the treatment milieu and clients' outcomes in each of three TC programs for substance abuse patients: Satori, The Family, and Quadrants. Satori, which was modeled on Jones' (1953) principles and was run primarily by professionally trained staff members, had moderate performance demands and sanctions and substantial emphasis on self-understanding and the open expression of anger. The Family had direct roots to Synanon and was run primarily by clients; it strongly emphasized confrontation, structure, self-help, and connection with family members and friends. In contrast, Quadrants, which was also run primarily by clients and paraprofessional staff, was much more loosely organized and allowed clients more freedom in personal conduct and expression.

Clients treated in Satori and The Family generally were doing better on substance use, work and school attendance, and criminal behavior criteria two years after treatment than were clients treated only in a five-day drug withdrawal program. In contrast, clients treated in Quadrants had improved less in these areas. Bale et al. (1984) thought that these clients' relative lack of improvement was related to Quadrants' emphasis on autonomy in the context of a lack of focus on self-understanding and less structure. Individuals with personality disorders may be more likely to improve in programs such as Satori and The Family, which are oriented toward dealing with personal problems in a clear and well-defined atmosphere.

Minnesota Model Programs

One of the most prevalent approaches to residential alcoholism treatment involves the Minnesota Model, which is based primarily on Alcoholics Anonymous (AA) principles and employs a relatively structured therapeutic community program to promote clients' personal responsibility for recovery, abstinence, and improvements in lifestyle (Cook, 1988). In a randomized trial, Keso and Salaspuro (1990) compared a Minnesota Model program with a traditional inpatient program. The Minnesota Model program was more supportive, expressive, and well-organized and oriented more toward understanding personal problems. Consistent with these findings, Minnesota Model patients were more likely to have continuing contact with AA after treatment and to be abstaining from alcohol at follow-up (26 percent versus 10 percent).

Outpatient Drug-Free Programs

The majority of adolescent clients with substance abuse problems are treated in outpatient "drug-free" programs. Aside from the fact that these programs tend to have few controls and relatively little structure, not much is known about these programs or how they affect their clients. To examine this issue, Friedman and Glickman (1986) asked clients and counselors to assess the treatment environment of thirty outpatient substance abuse programs for youth.

Programs that clients rated as more expressive and that staff rated as better organized and higher on practical and personal problem orientation showed a greater reduction in client-reported drug use from admission to discharge. Other program characteristics associated with better client outcomes included the provision of special services (such as vocational, birth control, school, and recreational services), the existence of an alternative school program, the use of specific types of treatment methods (such as crisis intervention and Gestalt therapy), and the presence of more experienced and better-trained staff. In general, these findings were replicated in two independent samples of clients and held after controlling for program differences in client populations (Friedman, Glickman, and Kovach, 1986b).

Friedman et al. (1986b) also found that the larger the discrepancy between client and staff perceptions of autonomy and staff control, the less successful the treatment outcome. Clients were less successful in programs in which they perceived staff as less encouraging of client autonomy and as exercising more control relative to the staff's perceptions of these dimensions. These discrepancies may reflect a lack of client-staff understanding and a feeling among the adolescent clients that staff lack trust in their maturity and decisionmaking.

Social Integration and Community Living Skills

In general, programs that encourage good relationships among clients and between clients and staff, are clear and well organized, and emphasize self-direction and self-understanding tend to facilitate clients' social integration and community living skills. Consistent with the idea that clients' levels of impairment may modify these associations, more disturbed and disabled clients may find it hard to adapt in more demanding, performance-oriented programs (see chapter 11).

Mentally Ill Clients in Group Homes

In an intensive, long-term study, Segal and Aviram (1978) focused on a sample of 499 sheltered care residents and the managers of the 234 facilities in which they lived. Clients who saw their program as more involving and well organized were less anxious, had fewer psychiatric symptoms, and were more satisfied with the program. Moreover, there were program-level associations between the quality of interpersonal relationships and the emphasis on personal growth goals and clients' participation in activities in the facility (internal social interaction) and activities in the community (external social integration). There also was a positive association between client-manager congruence in the relationship and personal growth areas and internal social integration (Segal, Everett-Dille, and Moyles, 1979).

The COPES was used to describe an ideal treatment environment as one that is involving and supportive, clearly organized, independence-fostering, oriented toward dealing with practical and personal problems, and conducive to the open expression of anger. The extent to which the program resembled this ideal environment was a strong predictor of clients' social integration in the facility. Among less disturbed or symptomatic clients, the ideal treatment environment was also associated with external social integration; that is, clients' participation in activities in the community. Among more severely disturbed or symptomatic clients, however, the ideal treatment environment seemed to insulate clients by promoting social integration in the facility but not integration into the community.

Long-term outcomes of support and performance expectations. Positive group home treatment environments, such as those that are supportive and client centered, may or may not enhance clients' long-term community outcome. To examine the role of supportive and high expectation residential care programs in the development of residents' social networks, Segal and Holschuh (1991) conducted a ten-year follow-up of 234 of the sheltered care residents who participated in Segal and Aviram's (1968) study. More than 75 percent of these individuals had schizophrenic disorders.

Highly supportive residential care environments were associated with a greater likelihood ten years later that the client would exchange emotional or instrumental support with another individual. In contrast, clients who lived in a high expectation environment, as measured by an emphasis on the development of social and work skills, ten years later had smaller social networks and less likelihood of exchanging emotional or instrumental support with members of their network. Thus, among relatively disturbed clients, more supportive facilities with fewer performance expectations contributed to the development of long-term supportive social networks. These findings imply that a supportive environment can contribute to clients' abilities to form and maintain relationships; they also raise a caution about the potential long-term negative impact of high performance expectations on severely impaired individuals.

Client empowerment and mastery. One prime motivation underlying the relocation of mentally ill individuals from hospital to community facilities is to reduce clients' institutional dependency. To examine the implementation of this goal, Segal and Moyles (1979) used selected COPES items to develop a Client Management Scale to tap the extent to which responsibility for decision making in group homes is placed with the resident (client centered) or with the facility manager (management centered). Dependency was measured by how much residents felt obligated to the manager, whether the resident wanted to stay in the home for a long period of time, and whether the resident believed that there were significant obstacles to leaving residential care. As expected, management-centered homes produced a pattern of client dependency, whereas client-centered homes did not.

From a broader perspective, a client-centered management style can contribute to clients' empowerment, especially when clients share programmatic responsibility with staff, have their ideas taken seriously, and are encouraged to make their own decisions. Rosenfield (1992) used COPES item to assess empowerment in a client-run psychosocial rehabilitation program based on the Fountain House model. She found that an empowerment approach to treatment and the provision of specific services, such as vocational rehabilitation services that educate clients about what to expect and how to act in the workplace, financial services directed toward securing economic resources, and groups that emphasized self-help and self-reliance were positively associated with clients' quality of life.

In an additional analysis, Rosenfield (1992) found that the empowerment approach and these services enhanced clients' sense of mastery, which, in turn, contributed to their quality of life. Clients' who received more services that helped to structure their free time also reported better quality of life; this association was independent of clients' sense of mastery. These findings imply that services that empower clients have positive effects on clients' life satisfaction by increasing their sense of mastery. In contrast, services that provide structure may enhance clients' satisfaction because they provide a sense of purpose or direction. By suggesting mechanisms through which services work, this type of conceptual analysis enhances our understanding of the potential links between program characteristics and clients' outcomes.

Developmentally Disabled Clients in Group or Foster Family Care

To evaluate the role of community residential facilities in the care of developmentally disabled adults, Willer and Intagliata (1984) studied individuals who were discharged from institutional care and were placed in one of 109 group homes or one of 229 foster family homes. Group homes were assessed with the COPES and foster family homes with the Family Environment Scale (FES; Moos and Moos, 1994a). The FES is conceptually comparable to the COPES in that it assesses relationship, personal growth, and system maintenance dimensions; one aspect of personal growth involves the family's level of social integration as reflected by it's cultural, recreational, and religious orientation. Clients were followed after two years or more in community placement; the baseline values of the outcome criteria were controlled in analyses that examined the influence of community facilities on clients' behavior.

In general, group homes that were involving, encouraged residents to take responsibility for themselves, and emphasized practical orientation enhanced residents' self-care and community living skills, social interaction, and use of community resources. Group homes that fostered the open expression of anger in a relatively structured context (that is, they tended to play down autonomy) facilitated control of maladaptive behavior among their residents. Overall, group homes that engage clients in the program and that set relatively high expectations for performance are most likely to facilitate clients' social functioning and adaptive behavior (see also Willer and Intagliata, 1981).

Clients in cohesive foster family homes that were oriented toward personal growth also showed better outcomes. Specifically, clients in homes that emphasized family social integration, as reflected by involvement in cultural and recreational activities and moral-religious orientation, developed more proficient self-care skills, interacted more with friends and relatives, and made more use of community resources. Clients in cohesive homes showed more control of their maladaptive behavior. In contrast, when the care providers were overprotective and controlling, clients showed fewer self-care and community living skills.

Clients' Perceptions and Community Adaptation

Some research has identified an association between clients' perceptions of a treatment program and their adaptation in the community. Specifically, clients who appraise a program more positively may be better integrated into the program and derive more benefit from it. Fischer (1979) noted that alcoholic clients who saw their program as clearer and oriented more toward self-understanding and the open expression of anger reported longer periods of abstinence and less frequent and shorter drinking bouts 10 weeks after discharge. Similarly, alcoholic clients who saw their treatment program as more involving and oriented toward independence and self-understanding were less likely to be readmitted to the hospital within a six-month period after discharge (Slater and Linn, 1982–83). Other researchers have also found that clients who see their program as clearer, better organized, and oriented more toward personal growth experience better treatment outcome (Dauwalder, et al., 1978).

We extended these findings in our study of the outcome of residential treatment for alcoholism. Patients in five programs were assessed at intake, completed the COPES to describe the program treatment environment, and were followed 6-8 months later. Patients who perceived the treatment environment more positively, as indicated by higher scores on all COPES dimensions except anger and staff control, reported less alcohol consumption, less severe drinking problems, and less physical impairment at follow-up (Cronkite and Moos, 1978). These findings held after controlling for patients' demographic characteristics and functioning at intake to treatment.

We followed a subset of these individuals ten years after treatment entry. As expected, patients' treatment experiences while in the program were not related to any ten-year outcome index. However, even after controlling for their demographic characteristics and functioning at intake, patients who appraised their treatment outcome more positively consumed less alcohol and had fewer physical symptoms and less depression ten years later (Finney and Moos, 1992). Although the precise mechanisms remain to be determined, clients' perceptions of a treatment program may provide important information about their integration into the program and long-term posttreatment adaptation.

Treatment Environment and Adjustment in the Community

We have identified some general relationships between aspects of treatment environments and indices of in-program and community adaptation. In terms of our tripartite categorization, supportive and well-organized programs that have high performance expectations tend to have patients who are more satisfied and self-confident. Expectations in specific areas tend to promote consonant coping styles, such that supportive programs facilitate affiliation, programs that emphasize self-understanding enhance self-revelation, and structured programs contribute to patients' dependency.

In general, characteristics of the treatment environment that are associated with better in-program outcomes are also linked to better psychosocial functioning and integration in the community. Cohesive programs that are relatively well-organized and emphasize the personal growth dimensions, especially autonomy and practical and personal problem orientation, tend to mitigate clients' symptoms and contribute to their psychosocial functioning and self-care and community living skills. Programs that keep clients out of hospital focus on the personal growth areas, especially independence, self-understanding, and skills development, as well as on maintaining supportive relationships and a moderate level of structure. Moreover, clients who report more emphasis in these areas in their programs, which may reflect the formation of a therapeutic alliance and integration into treatment, tend to do better on these community adjustment criteria.

Some of the findings also imply that program structure is more important for more impaired and more impulsive patients. Thus, staff control is associated with schizophrenic patients' community tenure, with improvement in substance abuse patients' symptoms and psychosocial functioning, and with developmentally disabled individuals' control of maladaptive behavior. We focus more explicitly on the potential benefits of client-program matching in chapter 11.

11

Special Issues:
Client-Program Congruence and
the Health Care Workplace

The findings described in chapters 9 and 10 identify general associations between treatment environments and clients' outcomes; that is, between variables in panels III and IV and panel V of the conceptual framework (figure 1.1). However, there is some evidence that different client subgroups may respond differentially to program support, performance expectations, and structure. Specifically, clients who are functioning relatively well seem to do better in moderately structured programs that emphasize social interaction and have high expectations for performance. In contrast, more impaired clients fare better in highly structured programs that have more limited expectations for performance and the open expression of feelings.

In an early example of a study that examined the connections between specific aspects of treatment process and patients' in-program outcomes, Kellam and his coworkers (1967) focused on twelve admission units for acute psychiatric patients, most of whom had schizophrenic disorders. Patients in more supportive programs improved most on several of the criteria; patients in programs with more self-direction and less structure (labeled adult status) showed the least improvement. This finding is consistent with the idea that more severely ill patients do less well in programs that have high expectations for performance. In general, such patients show better outcomes in less demanding programs.

Models of Client-Program Congruence

Some models of person-environment matching suggest that functionally competent individuals are better able to adapt to environmental demands than are individuals with impaired functioning (Lawton, 1989). Viewed in these terms, high environmental demands should have more positive consequences for clients who are functioning well than for those who are functioning poorly. Accordingly, a self-directed social climate that has high performance expectations and relatively little structure would have the most benefit for functionally able clients.

In contrast, functional and mental impairment sets limits on more disturbed clients' adjustment and behavior. Clients with acute schizophrenic disorders often find interpersonal stimulation disturbing; cognitively impaired clients may find it hard to cope with a strong emphasis on self-direction and skills development. Programs that require clients to structure their own daily activities may also be too demanding for some individuals. As clients' cognitive and psychosocial skills improve, they should be able to cope with a more demanding and somewhat less structured setting.

Patients' Level of Disturbance and Program Expectations

In a series of studies in Norway, Friis (1980, 1981b) examined these issues with respect to in-program outcomes. First, Friis compared actual and preferred treatment environments for three groups of patients who varied in their levels of disturbance and functioning. Acutely ill nonpsychotic patients were the least impaired, acutely ill psychotic patients were moderately impaired, and long-term chronic patients were the most impaired. The programs for acutely ill nonpsychotic patients were higher on the relationship and personal growth dimensions and lower on staff control; that is, they were more involving, had relatively high performance expectations, and were moderately structured. The programs for long-term chronic patients generally had the lowest expectations for social interaction and performance, and the programs for acute psychotic patients were in-between.

Patients' preferences were roughly in line with these differences in the actual treatment environments, indicating a good match between the programs and patients' needs (Friis, 1980). The fact that staff members in these three sets of programs showed somewhat stereo-typed preferences led Friis to conclude that patients' preferences may provide better standards against which to assess program implementa-tion than staff members' preferences do.

Preferred programs for psychotic and nonpsychotic patients. On the basis of these findings, Friis (1981b) defined the preferred treat-ment setting for less disturbed (nonpsychotic) patients as high on the relationship and personal growth dimensions and moderate on staff control. He thought that preferred programs for more disturbed (psy-chotic) patients would be supportive and well organized and would play down the open expression of anger. Compared to medication-oriented programs, group-oriented programs for nonpsychotic patients were closer to his model for such patients. For psychotic patients, however, group-oriented programs were no more supportive or well organized than medication-oriented programs. They also emphasized the open expression of anger. Accordingly, Friis (1981b) concluded that a group orientation may create an effective therapeutic milieu for less disturbed patients but not for more disturbed patients (see also Vaglum, Friis, and Karterud, 1985).

In a subsequent extension of this work, Friis (1986a) evaluated thirty-five short-term psychiatric programs using a Good Milieu index obtained from patients' reports of how satisfied they were with the program and how much they liked the patients and staff. For programs in which most of the patients were less disturbed (nonpsychotic), the Good Milieu index was higher when there was more emphasis on involvement, autonomy, and clarity. For programs in which most of the patients were more disturbed (psychotic), however, the Good Mi-lieu index was higher when there was less emphasis on spontaneity and the expression of anger. These findings support the idea that thera-peutic milieus for nonpsychotic patients should be more involving and self-directed, whereas programs for psychotic patients ought to have relatively little emphasis on venting affect.

Importantly, for both groups of programs, the Good Milieu index was higher in supportive and well-organized programs that empha-sized the development of social and work skills. Thus, provided that the focus on organization is not unduly restrictive and that the expec-tations for skills development are flexibly matched to clients' abilities, these aspects of a treatment climate may be of general benefit for patients with quite different levels of cognitive and functional impair-ment.

Notwithstanding these findings, a highly involving program that strongly emphasizes self-direction and skills development may have detrimental effects on severely neurotic clients, even though they are nonpsychotic and may be functioning relatively well. In this vein, neurotic clients treated in a highly involving, self-directed, and task-focused community program were readmitted twice as frequently as those treated in a traditional medical model program (Lehman and Ritzler, 1976). The strong emphasis on autonomy in the community program may have persuaded such clients to seek more independent and demanding situations in the community, thereby placing themselves at higher risk for readmission. The fact that many neurotic clients are quite passive and dependent may have made them especially susceptible to the influence of the treatment milieu.

Self-disclosure, structure, and patients' impairment. Several projects have examined these issues with respect to patients' adaptation in the community. In a study of seventy-nine VA programs, Collins et al. (1985) followed about 4,600 patients at three months after discharge. The outcome criteria were patients' posttreatment global adjustment as rated by the patients themselves and by collaterals; patients' pretreatment adjustment was controlled. Programs with more open patient-staff interaction tended to have better patient outcomes. These programs allowed patients to address staff by their first names, enabled patients to express their anger openly, and placed less emphasis on tight organization and control. Patients in highly structured programs that restricted the expression of anger had poorer outcomes. Because most of the patients in these programs were not chronically or severely disturbed, these findings are consistent with our characterization of programs with high community tenure rates (chapter 10).

Better programs also had fewer socially isolated patients and a higher percentage of patients who were off the unit during the day, primarily because they were participating in an activity. In addition, these programs had more current magazines in the dayroom and did not have a separate room with a television set. Such a room encourages patients to watch television, which may enable them to withdraw from program activities and thus give them an excuse for not participating actively in treatment (Ellsworth et al., 1979).

Nursing staff in the better programs were more stable; that is, they were less likely to be rotated to different shifts. Stable shift assignments enable staff to play a more responsible role in patients' therapeutic and social activities and perhaps to have a stronger positive influence on patients (Collins et al., 1984).

Klass, Growe, and Strizich (1977) focused on a quite different population composed primarily (90 percent) of chronic schizophrenic patients who had an average of more than four prior hospital episodes. In one set of fourteen programs, patients who were treated in well-organized programs that discouraged them from expressing anger were less likely to be violent and to cause injuries while hospitalized. Patients treated in these programs also tended to spend more time in the community after discharge. The stable social structure in these programs may have provided a model to help some patients plan their daily activities and thus to adjust better in the community. Patients in a second set of seven programs that did not differ in their emphasis on organization or expressiveness also did not differ in outcome.

These findings are consistent with Kahn and White's (1989) ideas about how to structure milieu treatment approaches for schizophrenic patients. When in an acute psychotic episode, such patients are typically overreactive and unable to process information accurately. Accordingly, they need a highly supportive and structured environment that focuses on the development of a working alliance with staff and plays down interpersonal stimulation and performance demands. At this stage, it is important to orient patients, establish clear expectations and rules, develop set schedules, and define the limits of acceptable behavior.

In support of these ideas, Cohen and Khan (1990) found that acute schizophrenic patients improved more in a highly structured psychiatric intensive care unit that focused on reality orientation than on an open unit with more stimulation and group treatment. As patients improve, they can begin to attend low-demand activity groups and then progress to focused discussion groups and perhaps to counseling groups. Over time, patients develop a sense of mastery over the crisis, reestablish their social connectedness, and enhance their self-understanding.

Self-disclosure and clients' minority status. Although an emphasis on personal problem orientation and self-understanding typically is beneficial for clients who are functioning relatively well, it may have negative effects for clients who are in a minority in the program, such as women in many substance abuse programs. Thus, we found that higher levels of perceived personal problem orientation were associated with better six-month outcomes among men in alcoholism programs. These findings did not hold among women. Men may be more receptive than women to an emphasis on self-disclosure and the exploration of personal problems in male-dominated, group-oriented treatment settings. In this respect, more participation in group therapy was associated with less alcohol consumption at follow-up among men but with more consumption among women (Cronkite and Moos, 1984). Similarly, Po (1989) noted that women who reported more personal problem orientation in a coeducational substance abuse program did less well in the program.

Program structure and patients with personality disorders. Program structure may be especially important for patients with personality disorders, who often find it difficult to control their impulses. Lehman and Ritzler (1976) compared a community program and a program that followed a traditional medical model. The community program was more involving, self-directed, and task focused, but less well organized. Character disordered clients in the community program dropped out of treatment more frequently, which implies that high expectations for performance in the context of a more open atmosphere may not be a good match for clients who have a low tolerance for frustration and tend to act on their impulses.

Although moderate program structure may help to retain clients in treatment and contribute to better in-program outcomes, an emphasis on staff control may not facilitate outcomes in less well-structured community settings. Consistent with this idea, we found that clients who reported more staff control in an alcoholism program showed poorer six-month treatment outcome. Among men, higher staff control was associated with more alcohol consumption and physical symptoms at follow-up; among women it was associated with more depression and fewer social activities. Clients with substance abuse disorders who are not severely impaired may respond adversely to staff efforts to maintain control through enforcement of rules and scheduling of activities (Cronkite and Moos, 1984).

Patients' Self-Care Dependency and Program Resources

Nursing homes currently constitute the largest system of long-term care for chronic mentally ill individuals (Bootzin, Shadish, and McSweeny, 1989). However, clinicians and researchers have questioned whether mentally ill individuals should be cared for in nursing homes, which were designed for a different population. They argue that people with a history of mental illness have fundamentally different needs than people who have functioned satisfactorily for most of their lives (Talbott, 1988). Several studies support the idea that chronic mentally ill individuals who are not well enough to live outside of institutions may function better and be happier in mental hospitals than in nursing homes (Linn et al., 1985; Shadish et al., 1985).

Linn and her colleagues (1985) speculated that mentally ill patients who resided in community nursing homes deteriorated because the other residents were highly impaired and because of a lack of psychiatric training and high turnover among staff in these facilities. Poor physical facilities and lack of planned activities and services are additional characteristics of nursing homes that may help explain the relatively poor functioning of mentally ill people living in them. Furthermore, policies in nursing homes tend to be more flexible and may not provide enough structure to meet mentally impaired patients' needs.

To examine these issues, we focused on the connections between specific characteristics of psychiatric and nursing home programs and chronically mentally ill patients' outcomes and, more specifically, on whether any such connections were moderated by patients' dependency on others for self-care (Timko et al., 1993). Consistent with Linn et al.'s (1985) speculations, community nursing homes provided residents with more choice and control and more prosthetic and orientational aids than psychiatric programs did. However, the nursing homes had more impaired residents, a lower staff-resident ratio, less well trained and experienced staff, and more staff turnover.

The facility characteristics that differentiated community nursing homes from psychiatric programs were associated with mentally ill patients' outcomes. Patients in facilities where other individuals were functioning better showed more vigor; patients in facilities that provided more opportunities for independence reported more vigor and greater life satisfaction. These findings lend support to Linn and associates' (1985) speculation that the poorer functioning of the other residents in community nursing homes contributes to mentally ill patients' greater deterioration in health and mental status relative to patients in psychiatric programs. The positive relationship between autonomy and adaptive functioning confirms the idea that mentally ill people benefit from policies that contribute to empowerment and mastery (Rosenfield, 1992).

The extent to which some program characteristics were beneficial or harmful varied, depending on patients' dependency on others for self-care. One pattern of findings showed that some supportive physical features and services were resources for highly dependent patients but seemed to restrict more independent patients' adaptive functioning. Specifically, more prosthetic and orientational aids and more daily living assistance services were related to better outcomes, particularly more vigor, for highly dependent patients but to worse outcomes for independent patients. According to Lawton's (1989) model, these aids served as resources for dependent patients by creating a good match between the level of environmental demand and patients' functional status. In contrast, the aids may have created an environment that was too supportive, or too low in demand and challenge for independent patients.

The second pattern of findings showed that better trained staff and policies that provided residents with more control were resources for more independent patients. Giving independent patients input into determining facility policies reduced their withdrawal and apathy; it helped them to stay involved with other residents and with their surroundings. The presence of more competent staff enabled independent patients to feel more vigorous. Dependent patients responded differently. Policies encouraging resident control appeared to create too much of a demand for dependent patients, who became more withdrawn and apathetic. Moreover, the presence of more competent staff did not affect dependent patients' vigor (Timko et al., 1993).

These results show that chronic mentally ill patients in nursing homes or psychiatric programs may obtain some benefit from an environment with more functionally able peers and policies that provide residents with more control. Environmental demands, as reflected by policies that encourage self-direction and more competent staff who likely have higher performance expectations, also have more positive effects on more independent patients. In contrast, supportive physical features and services have more positive effects on more dependent patients.

Residents' Functional Abilities and Self-Direction

Many of our findings are consistent with the idea that functionally competent individuals are better able to take advantage of environmental opportunities for self-direction. In a set of studies in residential facilities for older adults, we examined this issue at both the program and the individual level of analysis. At the program level (N = 262 facilities), an emphasis on residents' self-direction was associated with better adjustment and more participation in activities in the community, and with less reliance on the services offered in the facility.

More important, residents' functional abilities moderated the relationship between a self-directed social climate and residents' adaptation. In facilities with relatively intact residents, an orientation toward independence was strongly associated with better adjustment and less reliance on the services provided by the program. An emphasis on independence also appeared to benefit adjustment among impaired resident groups, but it did not affect their involvement in facility-planned activities or use of health and daily living services (Moos and Lemke, 1994; chapter 8)

These results are consistent with a matching model in which better functioning residents are better able to take advantage of opportunities for autonomy and control. More competent resident groups show better adaptation when policies support personal control and the social climate emphasizes independence. These policy and social climate factors have some benefits for more impaired resident groups but are generally less salient for them.

The findings were conceptually comparable at the individual level of analysis (N = about 1,400 residents). In general, an emphasis on independence was associated with residents' greater involvement in informal activities in the facility and in the community. These relationships were stronger for more intact than for impaired residents. A self-directed social climate is strongly related to activity involvement among well-functioning residents. This association remains positive but weakens as residents' functional ability declines (Moos and Lemke, 1994; chapter 9).

Consistent with Friis' (1986a) findings in psychiatric programs, supportive aspects of the setting, such as a cohesive social climate and good organization, were associated with better in-program outcomes regardless of the group's or the individual's level of functioning. Also comparable to the findings on psychiatric patients, organization was somewhat more strongly associated with involvement in planned activities among more impaired individuals. The importance of supportive relationships and order seems to hold for different types of resident groups and across a broad range of individual functioning.

Actual-Preferred Program Congruence

Thus far, we have focused primarily on experts' criteria for patient-program matching, especially with respect to patients' level of impairment and program expectations and structure. Another approach is to consider clients' preferences and their own judgments about how well they fit into specific programs.

In an application of this approach, family care residents who saw their home as more similar to their preferred home were more satisfied with the home and rated it as being of higher quality (Nevid, Capurso, and Morrison, 1980). Residents who saw the home as more similar to their preferred home in the areas of support, spontaneity, self-direction, practical orientation, and structure were rated by their caretakers as better adjusted to the home, functioning better socially, and showing less overt psychotic and problem behavior, and as likely to adjust better in the community in the future.

Another way to assess congruence, is to ask individuals to rate their needs and their environment on a set of commensurate dimensions. Coulton and her colleagues (1984a) used this procedure in a follow-up of individuals who were discharged from psychiatric hospitals into community care homes. Social workers rated clients' functioning at discharge from hospital; community care staff rated clients' functioning again after three months in the home.

When environmental demands were too strong, that is, when the expectations for autonomy and the development of social and work skills exceeded clients' capabilities, they showed less stability in functioning over time. Similarly, when clients' needs for privacy and self-understanding were not met, their functioning tended to decline. With respect to organization and control, clients in homes that had either more or less structure than they needed showed less stable functioning.

Coulton et al. (1984b) also found a connection between lack of client-program congruence and readmission to hospital. Clients who were in community care homes that had more emphasis on autonomy and self-understanding than they could handle were more likely to be readmitted. When programs emphasize performance expectations in specific areas, clients who cannot or will not meet them may be viewed as uncooperative, become more disturbed, and be more likely to be ejected from the community.

Clients in homes that allowed less spontaneity than they needed were also more likely to be readmitted. An expressive client may cause problems in a home where the norm is quiet acceptance and thus the client may be judged as disruptive or noncompliant.

Some aspects of client-program incongruence can stimulate a creative tension that promotes personal growth. Thus, clients who showed more self-understanding and less expressiveness than required in the home were more likely to remain in the community. These clients may have been dissatisfied by their interactions with clients and caretakers in the home, searched out relationships with other individuals, and thereby enhanced their social networks and psychosocial functioning. Moreover, as Segal and Aviram (1978) noted, clients who fit in well with a stagnant environment make little progress toward effective functioning in the community.

Matching Treatment Climates and Clients' Personal Resources

The studies we have reviewed show that performance expectations and program structure seem to affect clients differently, depending on their level of impairment. More intact clients react more positively in moderately structured programs that have more emphasis on self-direction, skills development, and self-understanding, whereas more disturbed clients prefer more structure and less emphasis on performance, especially self-disclosure. Clients who are functionally intact but who have problems controlling their impulses, such as many clients with character disorder and substance abuse problems, also are likely to experience better in-program outcomes in highly structured settings.

These findings, most of which are based on studies of psychiatric patients, generally are consistent with information drawn from studies matching alcoholic clients to treatment (Mattson et al., 1994). Structured, behaviorally oriented training in interpersonal and coping skills appears to work best for high-risk alcoholic clients who are less well educated, more anxious and impulsive, and/or have more severe psychiatric symptomatology. In contrast, low-risk clients who are better educated, less anxious and impulsive, and have few psychiatric symptoms seem to do better in more open interpersonally oriented treatment that emphasizes self-disclosure and the expression of feelings. Also consistent with the findings on psychiatric patients, conceptually more mature alcoholic clients may do better in less structured treatment settings.

The Health Care Workplace

An intervention program is not only a treatment setting for clients; it is also a work environment for health care staff. To develop an effective treatment setting, the work climate should satisfy staff. In this section, we consider the impact of the health care workplace on the treatment environment and on staff members' morale and performance.

There appear to be some special problems in the workplace in health care facilities. Compared to employees in other work settings, health care staff report less job involvement and less support from coworkers and supervisors. Moreover, many health care work settings are lacking in autonomy and clarity and are characterized by high work demands and supervisor control (Moos, 1994c). Staff in many programs engage in complex and anxiety provoking tasks, are not adequately prepared for their role, lack effective guidelines and supervision, and function in multidisciplinary teams in which they are not well accepted (Allen, 1993). Such difficult work conditions may contribute to a less supportive or well-organized treatment program and to low staff morale and impersonal care.

The Work Environment and Staff Morale

Morale among health care staff is higher in work settings in which co-worker relationships are open and supportive, the job is clear and well planned, and supervisors are flexible. When the workplace is supportive and clear and emphasizes independence and task orientation, staff members tend to feel they are accomplishing more at work and to report less emotional exhaustion and alienation (for a review, see Moos, 1994c). When high work demands occur in a setting that lacks cohesion and support, staff members report more emotional exhaustion and alienation. Co-worker and supervisor relationships may be especially strongly associated with job satisfaction among mental health staff because the quality of interpersonal relationships is a salient aspect of their work.

In a study of long-term care facilities, we found that staff members' perceptions of the work milieu were strongly associated with their job morale and performance. Staff who characterized their workplace as more involving and supportive, as more independent and clear, and as having fewer work demands were more satisfied with their job and less inclined to leave it. In general, these staff members also had fewer physical symptoms and were less depressed. These findings held at a follow-up about 8 months later, even when initial job morale and performance scores were controlled (Schaefer and Moos, 1993, 1996).

It is important to recognize that the work climate may vary extensively in different programs or divisions in a hospital. According to Starker's (1989) findings in a large urban VA medical center, acute inpatient units had high work demands and, because they were located in a new building, high physical comfort. Intermediate and long-term care units had the least work demands and, because they were located in older barracks-style buildings, low physical comfort. A small satellite outpatient clinic offered the most positive workplace; it was involving, cohesive, supportive, and clear. These findings emphasize the need to assess the work climate at the program level.

The Workplace and the Treatment Climate

By enhancing staff members' job morale and performance, a positive work milieu may enable staff to develop a better treatment environment, which, in turn, may be associated with better patient outcomes. According to O'Driscoll and Evans (1988), when staff saw the workplace as involving, cohesive, and oriented toward independence, they reported more involvement in the treatment milieu and patients reported more emphasis on self-understanding. In this vein, Meier (1983) identified a link between counselors' appraisals of the support they enjoyed in their work and the extent to which they encouraged their clients' independence.

In three residential cottages for emotionally disturbed youth, Johnson (1981) found that cohesion among staff members was associated with more support, self-direction, and practical and personal problem orientation in the treatment environment. Staff cohesion was also associated with lower levels of staff control in the treatment program. Similarly, Stirling and Reid (1992) found that a staff training program designed to encourage clearer communication and more problem-solving behavior among nurses resulted in residents viewing their environment as more supportive and self-directed, in an increase in their perceptions of control, and in improvements in their self-confidence.

In a study of more than 300 staff members in fifteen substance abuse treatment programs, Kyrouz and Humphreys (1996) identified some important links between the work and treatment climate. More supervisor support in the workplace was associated with more involvement and support in the treatment milieu. More managerial control in the workplace was associated with more emphasis in the treatment program on staff control and less on patient autonomy. Taken together, these findings suggest that there may be some direct "spillover" from the work to the treatment climate.

The Treatment Climate and Staff Morale

There are at least two related processes through which the treatment environment may be associated with staff members' job-related functioning. One possibility is that positive aspects of the workplace contribute to staff morale, which, in turn, enhances the treatment milieu. Another possibility is that there is a more direct relationship: Conditions that contribute to making the setting a positive environment for patients, such as a supportive and self-directed treatment climate, may also improve staff morale, perhaps because staff in such programs are providing treatment that is consistent with their values.

Consistent with the idea that there is a direct relationship between the treatment environment and staff morale, Dorr, Honea, and Pozner (1980) found that nurses who appraised the therapeutic climate of their program as more involving, supportive, clear, well organized, and oriented toward developing clients' work and social skills were more satisfied with their job. Similarly, in two outpatient programs for adolescents, counselors who reported more program support were more satisfied with their work (Fairchild and Wright, 1984). In contrast, staff members in hospital programs who thought that their program lacked clarity and organization and was high on anger experienced more anxiety (Friis, 1991). Programs that lacked support and clarity had more staff turnover (Friis, 1986b).

It is important to recognize that staff members are much less likely than are clients to react positively to program structure, especially when their latitude for decisionmaking is curtailed. Accordingly, Waxman, Carner, and Berkenstock (1984) found that nursing home aides who saw their units as highly organized and structured had high turnover rates. Aides who reported a more loosely organized administration and less rigid control had a lower turnover rate, perhaps because they enjoyed more autonomy. These findings are consistent with a matching model in which more competent individuals (staff members in this instance) prefer more control. More broadly, there likely is a reciprocal association between the treatment milieu and staff turnover; a more stable staff group may contribute to a more flexible treatment milieu.

Social Climate and Staff Functioning in Facilities for Older Adults

We have also focused on these issues among staff members in congregate facilities for older adults. Specifically, we examined the program-level (N = 262 facilities) links between the facility social climate and two measures of staff performance: observers' ratings of staff functioning and staff turnover. We controlled for the level of care and indices of workload as reflected by residents' social resources and functional abilities.

Facilities that were more cohesive, well organized, and oriented toward residents' self-direction had better functioning staff. Poorly organized facilities in which staff reported more conflict had higher staff turnover. Lack of group cohesion and interpersonal conflict appear to interfere with the quality of staff performance and their motivation to continue working in a facility. Of course, these factors are likely to be mutually reinforcing. Staff are more satisfied when they work in a supportive and predictable setting, and, as we saw earlier (chapter 8), better staff functioning may contribute to a supportive and self-directed treatment climate.

Earlier, we emphasized the importance of configural analyses of social climate factors; that is, of considering key aspects of the social environment in conjunction with each other. As a case in point, we studied a sample of nursing homes and found that the influence of organization varied in line with associated levels of cohesion and self-direction. Specifically, staff functioning was higher and staff turnover lower in programs that balanced order and predictability with staff and resident input (Brennan and Moos, 1990). In the context of harmonious relationships among staff and a climate of independence, organization tends to be appraised as enhancing clarity and facilitating shared goals and activities. Without cohesion and self-direction, however, an emphasis on organization may be experienced as restrictive and controlling.

Enriching the Work Environments of Health Care Staff

These findings imply that work and treatment climates may mutually reinforce each other and that both can have consequences for staff members as well as for clients. Where relationships are supportive and the workplace is flexibly organized, staff members experience higher morale, perform better, and are more likely to stay in their job. A decentralized or participative organization in which management seeks input from staff members seems to improve staff functioning and to facilitate individualized patterns of care. In turn, a social climate that emphasizes clients' self-direction appears to be beneficial for both clients and staff. Supportive and self-directed work and treatment environments may have beneficial consequences for each other and for staff members' morale and clients' adaptation.

Monitoring changes in work environments. In a process that is comparable to the action-oriented projects that have been conducted in treatment programs (chapters 3 and 6), program directors and evaluators can use information about the work climate to monitor and plan organizational change. For example, Wilderman and Mezzelo (1984) examined the effects on work climate of changing a community mental health center from a consultation model to a direct-service model. In the new mode of service delivery, staff spent more time with clients and less with their colleagues and had more regularity and structure in the work setting. Staff reported increases in job clarity and managerial control, but also a decline in staff cohesion, probably because staff members spent much less time with each other.

Quality Assurance (QA) programs are being widely instituted in health care settings, but little is known about how they affect staff morale. To examine this issue, Sinclair and Frankel (1982) compared two outpatient mental health programs. They selected one unit of each program to participate in QA activities and designated the other unit as a control. Contrary to their concern that QA activities might lower morale, staff members did not develop a more negative view of the work environment. In fact, staff in the QA group reported a rise in supervisor support and a decline in managerial control. Staff members who provided higher quality services saw the work climate as more cohesive and independent and less demanding (for additional examples, see Moos, 1994c).

One area in which more information is needed involves the way in which the organization of nursing services affects the work environment. In primary nursing, each nurse is responsible for the care of specific patients; in team and functional nursing, however, each nurse performs specific delimited tasks for a group of patients or for all patients on a unit. According to Thomas (1992), staff members in primary nursing programs report more support and autonomy than their team and functional nursing counterparts do. Being accountable for specific patients may enhance nurses' independence and relationships with coworkers and supervisors. These finding suggest that more emphasis on primary nursing might enhance staff morale.

Reducing work stressors. The assessment and feedback process can provide staff members and managers with information about the work climate and increase communication among them. It can be used to diagnose problems in a work group, identify work groups at risk for organizational dysfunction, facilitate team building, and plan and evaluate a change program. Tommasini (1992) found that information about the work climate enabled a staff support group led by a psychiatric liaison nurse specialist to raise clarity and management control closer to the levels the staff members preferred. A staff support group may also lead to an improvement in the treatment milieu (Amaral, Nehemkis, and Fox, 1981).

We found that the assessment and feedback process helped to identify and reduce work stressors among staff in an intensive care unit. Staff reported a lack of clarity and organization in the work milieu and relatively low co-worker cohesion and supervisor support. Group discussion of these findings helped to target problem areas and guide the staff in developing solutions, which included clarifying specific areas of individual responsibility and establishing regular meetings between nurses and physicians. Staff subsequently felt that the work climate improved, as shown by increases in job involvement and co-worker cohesion, more staff autonomy and clarity, and more emphasis on innovation. Staff morale and the quality of patient care also improved (Koran et al., 1983).

We have shown how to conceptualize and assess hospital and community program treatment environments, and how to use the resulting information to monitor and improve programs and measure the level of program implementation. In addition, we have reviewed research on the determinants and outcomes of treatment climates. In the next chapter, we highlight the key conclusions and describe directions for the future.

12

Implications for Treatment and Program Evaluation

In this chapter, we summarize the empirical work and discuss implications for program directors and evaluation researchers; we also offer ideas for more conceptually based evaluations of psychiatric and substance abuse treatment programs. After reviewing the findings on the determinants and outcomes of treatment environments, we cover some future trends, including a stronger focus on linking program characteristics and treatment outcomes, models and episodes of care, clients' life contexts and the generalization of treatment effects, and theory-based treatment evaluation.

We conceived our work as an integration of several lines of investigation. The initial conceptual basis of the research arose from studies indicating that individual behavior is sensitive to the context in which it occurs. The philosophy of moral treatment and its apparent beneficial effects, the link between program social structure and patients' symptoms, and the concept of the therapeutic community, are all based on the assumption that social context influences individuals' cognition and behavior. Comparative program evaluations have also shown how distinctive treatment environments can impel personal change.

To guide our work, we formulated a conceptual model to examine treatment programs and their influence on clients. The model encompasses objective program characteristics such as policies and services; clients' personal characteristics, including their symptoms and level of impairment; the treatment environment; and clients' in-program and community adaptation (figure 1.1). The model depicts the interplay between clients and treatment programs and can be generalized to focus also on staff. Because we thought that these ideas applied to hospital and community programs, we focused on treatment environments in both of these loci of care.

Characterizing Treatment Environments

We formulated parallel procedures to measure the treatment climate of hospital and community programs by asking clients and staff about the usual patterns of behavior in their program. We were compelled by the logic that individuals' behavior is shaped by the environment as they perceive it. In addition, we wanted to be able to compare clients and staff members' views of treatment environments, as well as to contrast individuals' perceptions of actual and preferred programs.

We developed the Ward Atmosphere Scale (WAS) to depict the treatment environment of hospital programs and the Community-Oriented Programs Environment Scale (COPES) to depict the treatment environment of community programs. We initially surveyed more than 200 hospital programs and seventy-five community programs in the United States and the United Kingdom. The psychometric data showed that the WAS and COPES subscales have adequate internal consistency and test-retest reliability, discriminate significantly among treatment programs, and are only moderately interrelated. We also found that the social climate of programs that have a consistent treatment philosophy can be quite stable over relatively long intervals, even though there is complete turnover in the client population.

Conceptually, the WAS and COPES subscales fall into three common underlying domains. Involvement, support, and spontaneity measure the quality of interpersonal relationships. Autonomy, practical orientation, personal problem orientation, and anger and aggression assess the strength of performance expectations in four personal growth areas. Order and organization, clarity, and staff control reflect the level of structure in a program. This framework helps to understand the characteristics and outcomes of treatment programs and to link the findings to research in related areas, such as how psychotherapy and self-help groups influence patients and how the health care workplace affects staff.

Clients' and Staff Members' Perceptions

On average, clients and staff seem to perceive treatment programs somewhat differently. Compared with clients, staff consistently report that programs are more involving, supportive, and expressive, and have more emphasis on each of the personal growth areas. Staff also tend to report more clarity but less staff control. In general, these findings hold in psychiatric and substance abuse programs, as well as in hospital and community programs. Staff members probably present a more positive picture of treatment programs than clients do because they are responsible for organizing the programs and thus are more likely to understand them and to experience and emphasize their better aspects.

Clients' and Staff Members' Preferences

One way to assess whether a program is well implemented is to compare it with it's clients' and staff members' preferences. Information about preferences also helps consultants develop specific plans about how to change a program. Accordingly, we developed Ideal Forms of the WAS and COPES to enable clinicians and program evaluators to assess clients' and staff members' ideas about actual and optimal programs on common dimensions.

Clients' and staff members' overall preferences are relatively similar, although staff prefer somewhat more emphasis on each of the relationship and personal growth dimensions and somewhat less focus on staff control. These differences are comparable to those that exist in clients' and staff members' perceptions of actual programs. They suggest that staff members' roles and responsibilities shape loftier goals for ideal programs as well as more positive perceptions of actual programs.

The Diversity of Treatment Programs

Our findings show that hospital and community treatment programs are quite diverse. Nevertheless, there are some prototypic sets of programs. Traditional therapeutic community programs emphasize self-direction, self-disclosure, and the open expression of anger and play down organization and control. Modified therapeutic community programs for substance abuse patients also emphasize self-direction and self-disclosure; however, they are much more carefully structured. In contrast, social learning and vocational rehabilitation programs play down self-understanding and emphasize instead the development of clients' work and social skills in a moderately supportive and highly structured context.

Another way to search for general types of treatment environments is to conduct empirical cluster analyses. We used this procedure to identify six common types of hospital and community programs: therapeutic community, relationship oriented, action oriented, insight oriented, control oriented, and undifferentiated. These findings show that the locus of care does not define the treatment climate: hospital programs can be supportive and self-directed and community programs can be highly structured and custodial. More important, a substantial proportion of both hospital and community programs are not well implemented with respect to the quality of relationships or a balanced emphasis on clients' personal growth.

Program Implementation

The assessment of treatment implementation is the first step in understanding the content of treatment and in carefully studying the treatment process. We described three main ways to gauge how well a program is implemented: comparison with normative standards, comparison with clients' and staff members' preferences, and comparison with experts' judgments. Some programs may be well implemented with respect to all three of these sets of criteria, but, more commonly, a program may meet or exceed normative standards but not yet be optimal in terms of its' clients' or staff members' desires.

Implementation assessments are of considerable practical value. For example, such assessments enable evaluators to find out whether programs with contrasting professed treatment goals actually develop treatment environments consistent with these goals. They can also identify programs that may be ineffective because they are well implemented according to staff but not according to clients.

Program managers often need to make key resource allocation decisions, such as whether or not to try and establish a milieu-oriented program in a specific administrative context, such as a short-stay admissions unit or a forensic hospital. Implementation assessments have shown that milieu-oriented programs can function in these contexts, but that they tend to be less supportive and more structured than typical therapeutic community programs. In addition, due to their complex social system and dependence on a stable staff group, even well-implemented therapeutic community programs may be evanescent and subject to decay. Accordingly, before trying to develop such programs, it is important to be sure that there is sufficient administrative support to maintain them.

Our implementation assessment of residential alcoholism programs, which distinguished the programs in ways that were consistent with their treatment orientations, illustrated several important points. For example, it showed that required participation in treatment activities does not necessarily ensure an involving, supportive treatment environment and that an adequate amount of treatment may not lead to positive treatment quality. Conversely, programs that are brief and rely on very few psychosocial treatment components can create an effective treatment climate, as was true of an aversion conditioning program we studied. We also learned that a program managed by nonmedical staff can develop an engaging, self-directed social climate, as shown by a Salvation Army program in our sample.

Another application of implementation assessment is to examine the influence of staff training and experience on the treatment environment. In this vein, we compared programs that had professionally trained staff with programs that had only paraprofessional staff. These programs did not differ in the relationship areas; however, programs with professionally trained staff placed more emphasis on clients' personal growth, whereas programs with only paraprofessional staff placed more emphasis on program structure. By identifying differences in implementation that are linked to staff training, these findings highlight the value of an effective mix of professional and paraprofessional staff in a program.

Community versus Hospital Programs

Although there is considerable overlap in the quality of the treatment environment in hospital and community programs, there also are some consistent overall differences. Perhaps because clients are less acutely disturbed and not in a crisis situation, community programs for mentally ill individuals tend to be more supportive and expressive, more oriented toward self-direction, and clearer and better organized than are hospital programs. In general, these findings hold for substance abuse programs, although the differences are less extensive. Contrary to the idea that hospital programs necessarily are more custodial, however, community programs can be higher on staff control.

It is important to recognize that nonresidential outpatient programs, which may be less restrictive, are not necessarily more effective than community residential programs. Although they typically are more expensive, the full-time, live-in nature of residential programs may provide much more support and structure, as well as a transitional setting that both protects clients and offers the opportunity for them to learn and practice new social and vocational skills.

Our findings reflect a dramatic change from the situation in the past, when many community programs were newly developed and relatively poorly staffed, and provided few if any treatment services. As proponents of the community mental health movement envisioned more than forty years ago, the focus of ongoing treatment seems to have moved from the hospital to the community. Provided that continuing supportive services are available, this shift should be associated with better treatment outcomes.

Monitoring and Improving Programs

According to our own and other evaluators' findings, the WAS and COPES can be used to monitor program change and to guide the process of improving existing programs and developing new ones.

Monitoring Program Change

Treatment programs are continually changing, often by chance and sometimes by design. When program modifications are carefully monitored, we can enhance our understanding of the process of change and learn how to counteract potential problems, such as a temporary decline in clients' perceptions of program clarity. Effective implementation of a change in a program's overall treatment goals should eventually result in a high level of clarity and organization and, because of increased communication between clients and staff about new program policies and procedures, a rise in the quality of interpersonal relationships.

Changes in the personal growth dimensions are linked somewhat more closely to the specific changes in staff members' performance expectations for clients. When custodial or medically oriented programs are reoriented toward therapeutic community principles, the focus on personal problem orientation and the open expression of anger tends to rise. In contrast, the implementation of a social learning or behavior modification program is most likely to enhance practical orientation and autonomy. We also found that an individualized case management program resulted in a rise in autonomy. These findings can help a program evaluator identify when programmatic changes result in expected changes in the treatment environment, and, if they do not, to take corrective action.

Program monitoring can also identify unexpected effects of new policies or procedures. Although a continuous care unit would be expected to have a more supportive and active treatment climate than admissions or predischarge units that are part of a two-step model of care, in one evaluation the continuous care unit was less supportive, less self-directed, and less well organized. Subsequent analysis showed that the continuous care model enhanced staff morale, but that a shorter hospital stay detracted from this model's positive effects on the treatment environment and clients' long-term adjustment. Another example is the finding that, contrary to expectations, patients rated staff members as more helpful and supportive when they wore uniforms than when they wore street clothes.

Promoting Program Improvement

In a sequence of action-oriented assessment, feedback, and intensive discussion and planning, program evaluators can educate staff about their program's treatment climate and motivate them to improve it. For example, the staff in a psychiatric unit of a general hospital used the WAS to describe the program and, working with a consultant, to create a more active treatment milieu. After the completion of the feedback and change process, patients saw a clearer, more supportive program that focused less on self-understanding and more on independence and the development of social and work skills. The underlying direction of the program remained stable, indicating that important changes can unfold within a consistent treatment philosophy.

A treatment environment cannot be changed toward a static ideal;

feedback and discussion of program-relevant information is a dynamic, ongoing process that may produce changes in both the actual and preferred treatment milieu. These changes may flow in both directions: changes in individuals' preferences may motivate changes in the program; in turn, changes in the program may alter individuals' preferences. In this vein, clients and staff members in a community residential center for youth reported that the overall treatment milieu was closer to their preferences after program modifications were made, but that they wanted less focus on self-disclosure and the expression of anger.

Several conclusions emerge from these and other comparable studies.

- An ongoing formative evaluation can help to make staff members more aware of the treatment climate and how it influences clients.
- Information about the treatment environment identifies problematic aspects of the program and helps clients and staff to understand that they can alter the program and to plan specific changes to do so.
- Attempts to change a program may have temporary negative effects, such as a decline in perceived support and clarity. To avoid such problems, staff need to spend more time with clients and clearly explain the new treatment goals and activities.
- Consultants can help staff make specific changes within a consistent treatment ideology; however, they can also plan more dramatic shifts in the basic direction of a program, such as from a psychodynamic to a rehabilitation orientation.

Determinants of Program Climate

Hospital and community programs vary widely in their treatment environments. To examine some of the reasons for such variations, we expanded our model to focus on the determinants of the treatment climate. Specifically, we focused on how the institutional context (factors such as ownership, size, and staffing), physical features, policies and services, and the aggregate characteristics of the residents and staff (the suprapersonal environment) influence the treatment environment.

With respect to institutional context, nonprofit programs and smaller and better staffed programs are more supportive and well-organized and have more emphasis on autonomy and practical and personal problem orientation. More physical amenities and space also contribute to a supportive and self-directed program, as do more resident control and clearer policies. More health and treatment services are specifically associated with more emphasis on clients' skills development and self-understanding.

The aggregate characteristics of the residents and staff in a program are also associated with the treatment environment. Programs with older, more mentally impaired clients tend to be less supportive and self-directed and less focused on practical and personal problem orientation. In contrast, when clients have more social resources and staff are more experienced and effective, programs tend to be more supportive and self-directed and more likely to emphasize self-understanding.

Overall, the institutional context and physical, policy, and suprapersonal factors appear to have mutually reinforcing influences on the type of social climate that emerges in a program. These findings can identify specific interventions that can contribute to a more supportive, resident-directed, and well-organized social climate. Thus, for example, program cohesion can be enhanced in a number of ways: by increasing social-recreational aids and space, by assigning staff teams to be responsible for specific groups of residents, by developing clearer policies that enable residents to participate more actively in facility decisionmaking, and so on. The findings can also help to understand and counteract unexpected effects on the treatment climate, such as when providing residents with more choice over their daily activities leads to a decline in support and organization.

Outcomes of Program Climate

Following the conceptual model, we focused on in-program outcomes, community adaptation, and client-program congruence. Overall, our findings show that high performance expectations and moderate structure have a positive influence on many clients, but that it is important to consider the match between the program climate and clients' abilities.

In-Program Outcomes

We identified some consistent relationships between characteristics of the treatment environment and clients' in-program outcomes. Clients in supportive and well-organized programs that have moderate to high performance expectations tend to be more satisfied and self-confident and to participate more in program activities. In contrast, programs that lack support and organization tend to have high dropout rates; clients who report less program focus on support and organization are more likely to drop out. Programs that are relatively structured and that emphasize clients' work and social skills tend to discharge clients quickly and efficiently.

The associations between the treatment environment and clients coping and interpersonal behavior are more delimited. Specific aspects of a program are linked to clients' initiatives in consonant areas: program involvement promotes clients' affiliation; personal problem orientation facilitates clients' self-revelation; a focus on aggression enhances clients' expression of anger; staff control elicits clients' compliance with program directives. These findings highlight the value of a supportive, well-organized treatment environment that is somewhat self-directed and sets moderate to strong performance expectations for clients. They also emphasize the more focused connections between specific program characteristics and clients' in-program behavior.

Adaptation in the Community

In general, aspects of the treatment environment that are associated with better in-program outcomes are also linked to better social and vocational functioning and integration in the community. Specifically, cohesive programs that are relatively well-organized and emphasize the personal growth dimensions, especially self-direction, skills development, and self-understanding, tend to mitigate clients' symptoms and contribute to their psychosocial functioning and self-care and community living skills.

Programs that keep patients out of the hospital focus on the personal growth areas, especially independence and work and social skills, as well as on maintaining supportive relationships and a moderate level of structure. Patients who report more emphasis in these areas in their programs, which may reflect the development of a therapeutic alliance and integration into treatment, tend to do better on community adjustment criteria.

Client-Program Congruence

Although there are consistent overall relationships between program characteristics and clients' outcomes, performance expectations and staff control seem to affect some clients differently, depending on their level of impairment. Better functioning clients react more positively in moderately structured programs that have more emphasis on self-direction, skills development, and self-understanding. More disturbed clients prefer more structure and less emphasis on performance, especially self-disclosure. One exception is that clients who are functionally intact but who have problems controlling their impulses are likely to experience better in-program outcomes in highly structured settings. Because program structure may not help such clients learn to control their impulses in real-life situations, however, it does not seem to be associated with better community adaptation among these clients.

Overly active stimulation and strong demands for independent functioning can lead to an exacerbation of symptoms and relapse among impaired clients who are pushed to the limit of their abilities. Some clients with more severe and chronic disorders are more likely to remain asymptomatic in a tolerant and supportive setting that permits them to remain uninvolved than they would in a setting that seeks to engage them in confrontation and self-disclosure. High performance expectations may lead to better outcomes for some clients, but they can also contribute to dissatisfaction and attrition among clients who are less motivated or less able to change.

These basic findings are consistent with the general conclusions of recent reviews of treatment outcomes among individuals with psychiatric and substance abuse disorders. According to Paul and Menditto (1992), more chronic and impaired clients do not have sufficient skills to benefit from more self-directed high demand programs. Acutely disturbed clients, such as those with schizophrenic disorders, are likely to be overstimulated by such programs, in part because they cannot readily comprehend program policies and procedures. Clients who have problems controlling their aggressive behavior also need more structured programs. Paul and Menditto (1992) conclude that more chronic patients do best in structured social learning programs that carefully match performance expectations to patients' current cognitive and behavioral skills (see also Halford and Hayes, 1991).

Future Trends

Over the past decade, evaluation researchers have obtained growing evidence that treatment for psychiatric and substance abuse disorders can lead to positive behavioral and psychosocial outcomes and to a reduction in the overall use of health care services (Langenbucher, 1994; Pallak et al., 1994). Specific types of psychological and behavioral interventions, including coping skills training, family counseling and education, and self-help groups such as Alcoholics Anonymous (AA), are consistently associated with a reduction in symptoms and improvements in psychosocial functioning (Finney and Monahan, 1996; Lipsey and Wilson, 1993; Seligman, 1995). Moreover, individuals who enter treatment tend to improve more than untreated individuals do and those who stay in treatment longer improve more than those with shorter episodes of care (Timko, Finney, and Moos, 1995).

As described earlier, three broad trends currently characterize mental health care. Spurred by health care reform and the specter of market competition, there is growing emphasis on evaluating the process and outcome of treatment, especially the relative benefits of different packages of treatment services. A second trend is to redirect treatment from a primary focus on acute inpatient care to less expensive modes, such as community residential care and case-managed outpatient care. These two changes have led to a third trend: more emphasis on continuity and coordination of care.

Taken together, our findings and these trends point to several sets of issues that program evaluators should address. One set of issues focuses on developing a better understanding of program characteristics and services and their connections to treatment outcomes among different client populations. A related set of issues is to consider integrated models and packages of care, such as specialty programs for clients with substance abuse and psychiatric disorders and episodes of care that encompass hospital and community treatment as well as formal and informal services. Another important issue is to examine the generalization of treatment effects in light of the characteristics of clients' actual life contexts. Finally, we need more information about the theory of treatment; that is, about specific treatment orientations and how they contribute to the proximal and long-term outcomes their proponents predict should occur.

Program Characteristics, Services, and Outcomes

Our findings identify at least two salient characteristics of treatment programs other than their social climate: treatment orientation, including specific program goals and activities, and program policies and services. We need more information about the underlying treatment orientations that characterize psychiatric and substance abuse programs, how these orientations reflect different models of care, and how they contribute to the treatment environment and treatment outcome. The main questions about policies and services are how to strike a workable balance between institutional order and individual freedom for different groups of clients and the extent to which enriched services actually contribute to better treatment outcomes.

Treatment orientations. The literature in psychiatric and substance abuse care describes different models of treatment, such as therapeutic community, psychodynamic, rehabilitation, social learning, and AA/twelve-step. Many clinicians believe that these models are especially appropriate for particular groups of patients. To better understand the specific treatment goals and activities that underlie these models, we developed a measure of treatment orientations for substance abuse programs, the Drug and Alcohol Program Treatment Inventory (DAPTI), which can be applied to inpatient and extended care programs, community residential programs, and outpatient and day hospital programs (Moos, Pettit, and Gruber, 1995a; Swindle et al., 1995).

The DAPTI and other such measures can be used to describe a program's underlying approach to treatment, to compare alternative models of treatment, to identify connections between contrasting models and the treatment climate, and to examine the continuity of hospital, community residential, and outpatient treatment not only in terms of specific providers but also in terms of actual processes of care. For example, because many clients are exposed to different models of care, we need to understand the combined influence of treatment in a social learning program preceded or followed by treatment in a twelve-step program. Taken together, information about the treatment environment and treatment orientation should provide a more integrated picture of hospital and community programs and how they influence clients' outcomes.

Policies and services. Treatment programs vary substantially in their policies and services, especially in terms of expectations for clients' functioning and acceptance of problem behavior, rules about clients' choice in activities of daily living and participation in program governance, and the provision of health and treatment services. Timko (1995) developed the Policy and Services Characteristics Inventory (PASCI) to assess these characteristics and to compare divergent programs, such as hospital with community programs and substance abuse with psychiatric programs. Compared with hospital programs, for example, community programs have higher expectations for clients' functioning, provide more formal mechanisms for clients to influence program policies, and offer clients more choice in their pattern of daily activities.

Comparisons such as these are becoming more important as clients move more quickly from acute inpatient to community residential care, especially because more impaired clients may not be able to adapt successfully in self-directed, high-demand community programs that are less tolerant of problem behavior. Measures such as the PASCI enable evaluators to examine the connections between policies and services and in-program and community outcomes for clients who vary in their levels of functioning and mental disturbance.

A number of other issues should also be pursued in more depth. One issue is the changing interplay of client and program characteristics as clients' improve and mature. We need to learn more about when to increase performance expectations and reduce structure as clients' symptoms abate. In addition, we should try to identify program characteristics that are positively associated with clients' in-program as well as their community outcomes. Another issue involves the potential detrimental effects of highly supportive, low demand programs, which may constrain clients' freedom and inhibit their personal growth. Highly cohesive programs that play down self-direction may narrow clients' search for relevant information and thereby reinforce their passivity and dependence.

Models and Episodes of Care

Two important developments in mental health care involve a growing number of conceptual models, such as those for clients with both psychiatric and substance abuse disorders and those for community-based systems of care, and an emphasis on managed care and the outcomes and costs of entire episodes rather than just specific components of care.

Program models for clients with dual diagnoses. Epidemiological studies have shown that more than 40 percent of individuals with an addictive disorder also have a psychiatric disorder within the same twelve-month interval; the lifetime co-occurrence of these disorders is more than 50 percent (Kessler et al., 1996). These comorbidity rates may be even higher among individuals in the treatment. Recognizing the sharp differences in models of psychiatric and substance abuse care, treatment providers are trying to develop integrated treatment approaches for these individuals (Drake et al., 1996; Schmidt and Weisner, 1993). The common elements of an emerging model of dual diagnosis treatment are careful assessment and differential diagnosis, staging of treatment to enhance motivation prior to initiating substance abuse counseling, a more tolerant environment with fewer and more relaxed program rules than is typical in most substance abuse programs, an avoidance of potentially addictive medications, and intensive case management and outpatient aftercare.

Compared with traditional substance abuse programs, Swindle et al. (1995) found that dual diagnosis programs had more emphasis on psychotropic medication and greater tolerance of medication noncompliance and relapse. More tolerance of problem behavior and the presence of twelve-step groups were associated with lower-than-expected readmission rates. Patients in programs with lower dropout rates, longer episodes of care, and more assertive outpatient psychiatric aftercare also did better than expected. Several other studies have shown that dual diagnosis patients do better in integrated than in parallel psychiatric and substance abuse care (Drake, et al., 1996).

This work provides some initial evidence linking conceptually relevant program characteristics to dual diagnosis patients' proximal and longer-term outcomes. Future studies should examine alternative models of dual diagnosis care, the links between these models and program characteristics, and the connections between these factors and patients' in-program and community outcomes. Such studies should also consider potential differential outcomes for clients with varying levels of impairment and varying psychiatric disorders.

Models of community residential care. As noted earlier, there is a growing trend to refer psychiatric and substance abuse clients for community residential care, in part because of its promise of greater effectiveness and relatively low cost compared with acute inpatient care. Accordingly, more information is needed about the main models of care in community residential facilities. In an initial approach to this issue, we identified three such models: psychosocial, supportive rehabilitation, and intensive treatment.

Compared with psychosocial and supportive rehabilitation models, an intensive treatment model had lower expectations for clients' functioning, offered clearer policies and more resident participation in facility governance, provided more daily living assistance services and social-recreational activities, and had more emphasis on medical and dual diagnosis treatment orientations. Unexpectedly, intensive treatment programs were no more likely than psychosocial programs to treat chronic clients or clients who had both psychiatric and substance abuse disorders (Moos, Pettit, and Gruber, 1995a). These findings show that there are contrasting models of community care, but that these models may not be well-matched to their clients' needs.

Clients treated in the three models of care varied somewhat in proximal and longer-term outcomes. Specifically, clients in intensive treatment programs were seen for longer episodes of residential care and were likely to obtain more intensive outpatient mental health aftercare. In each of the three treatment models, clients who had longer episodes of care were less likely to be readmitted for acute inpatient care. More research is needed to focus on how clients are selected for different models of community care and to examine the effects of these models and of the intensity of care on clients' outcomes.

Managed care and episodes of care. The emergence of managed care and capitated systems of reimbursement, in which health care organizations receive a fixed amount of funding for each individual under their care, is changing the nature of evaluation issues. Health care managers now want to know the outcomes and costs of clients' entire episodes of care, including mental health and medical care and hospital and community care. To address these questions, we will need to define and characterize not only specific programs and treatment components but also broader combinations or packages of services.

Cost analyses are an important aspect of this expanding model of evaluation research. By focusing not only on the effects of alternative services but also on the cost of resources needed to achieve them, such analyses can provide decision makers with important information (Yates, 1995). In this regard, Rosenheck, Frisman, and Gallup (1995) examined the relationship between several treatment components and the outcome of a program for homeless individuals with psychiatric and substance abuse disorders. The number of days in residential treatment was strongly linked to improvement; however, it was also more costly than other effective treatment components such as case management.

Because residential treatment and case management may lead to improvement in different domains, as was the case in Rosenheck et al.'s (1995) study, the implications of cost analyses may not always be clear cut. Nevertheless, cost analyses should enhance the practical benefits of outcome evaluations. An effort to identify the costs of services should increase the data available on clients' participation in specific treatment components, which will facilitate treatment implementation and treatment process analyses. An effort to identify the broader benefits of treatment may enhance the likelihood of an analysis of the impact of treatment on a diverse array of criteria, including clients' coping skills and community adaptation.

Clients' Life Contexts and the Generalization of Treatment Effects

Even though we have focused almost entirely on program characteristics here, we have noted the importance of clients' life contexts and their influence on clients' longer-term treatment outcome (Moos et al., 1990). In fact, formal and informal treatments may influence community outcomes only insofar as they either change clients' life contexts or provide clients with long-term skills that help them develop and maintain more benign life circumstances.

Social learning approaches try to strengthen clients' underlying social and role functioning skills and may be effective when clients actually employ these skills in their daily lives and are rewarded for doing so. Unfortunately this may not happen regularly in the natural community environment (Halford and Hayes, 1991). Psychodynamic approaches try to increase clients' self-understanding and open expression of affect, but again these characteristics may not be valued in many community settings, as Rapaport's (1960) evaluation of the Belmont therapeutic community revealed. Similarly, increasing clients' self-direction and empowerment may work in the long run only to the extent that these characteristics find a compatible niche in the community.

Other treatment approaches focus more directly on clients' community contexts. Family psychoeducation and family and marital systems treatments may work well because they change clients' long-term social environment in part by changing clients' and family members' cognitive and behavioral coping responses. Fairweather and colleagues (1964) idea of a community lodge in which clients are part of an integrated task group reflects the importance of creating a supportive community milieu, as does Azrin's (1976; Azrin et al., 1982) community reinforcement approach and, more generally, the development of community residential programs. Even more dramatically, AA and other self-help programs are based on the goal of creating an ongoing social network to support a pervasive and permanent change in an individual's life-style.

In a review of psychosocial treatments for alcohol use disorders, we noted that the most effective modalities included social skills training, self-control training, motivational counseling, behaviorally oriented marital treatment, and community reinforcement. There was also some evidence for the effectiveness of behavioral contracting, stress management training, and relapse prevention training (Finney and Moos, in press). Each of these modalities focuses primarily on enhancing the client's real-world skills in coping with everyday life circumstances, altering contingencies in the natural environment, and improving the match between the client's abilities and environmental demands. Less effective treatments such as individual counseling and psychoeducation do not tend to focus as explicitly or intensively on teaching clients' how to cope with their life circumstances outside the treatment situation.

In conducting future evaluations, we need to pay special attention to how program characteristics and services may impact on clients' life contexts and community-relevant coping responses. It is important to consider how formal and informal services may maintain changes in clients' social and vocational skills as well as how they can help to restructure clients' family, work, and social contexts in the community. (For an integrated way to assess these contexts, see Moos and Moos, 1994b.) The most active and powerful ingredients of treatment may be those that improve the match between clients' abilities and the environment's expectations.

Theory-Based Treatment Evaluation

By measuring characteristics of program processes and services, and by linking these indices to treatment outcome, program evaluators can make a contribution toward theory-based evaluation research. In this regard, Finney (1995) has described two general ways to use theoretical frameworks to guide treatment evaluation projects and thereby make them more explanatory. By specifying the mediators of treatment effects, program evaluators can focus on how or why a treatment does or does not work. By specifying the moderators of treatment effects, program evaluators can identify specific groups of clients for whom different treatments work especially well.

Morgenstern and his colleagues (1996) used a theory-driven approach to assess the specific processes that adherents of the Minnesota Model think mediate positive treatment outcome. These processes include acknowledging powerlessness over the substance use, belief in a higher power, endorsement of the disease model, and commitment to AA. Clients showed only small increases in their endorsement of these disease model processes; moreover, the strength of their beliefs in these processes was not linked to abstinence from substance use. Clients who had stronger beliefs in two common processes that are considered important by adherents of the Minnesota Model and other treatment approaches, commitment to a goal of abstinence and to avoiding high-risk situations, were more likely to remain abstinent. These findings show how a theory-driven examination of proximal change processes can help to identify the critical mediators of treatment outcome.

In addition to clarifying the proximal changes that may impel better long-term outcomes, it is important to specify more precisely the client and staff behaviors that foreshadow these changes. Paul (1987) has emphasized the need for a practical, decision-oriented assessment technology that identifies and describes clients' problems, monitors clients' progress on an ongoing basis, and helps clinicians plan clients' placement and treatment. To this end, Paul describes specific procedures that assess clients' problem behaviors and how staff members' treatment techniques influence these behaviors. When treatment process analyses identify potential mediators of change, such procedures can be used to help staff assess and learn how to influence these mediators.

There is growing consensus that program evaluations are most useful when embedded in a theoretical context—when an evaluation tries to explain or generate additional knowledge about treatment processes and their connections to in-program and longer-term outcomes. Because this approach embeds an evaluation in a theory of the treatment process and of the clients' disorder, it is more likely to identify sources of treatment failure and decay in treatment gains, to consider the role of life context factors in outcome, and to help formulate ways to improve treatment.

Advances in each of the areas we have discussed should help to improve the quality of psychiatric and substance abuse programs and thereby contribute to enhancing clients' adaptation and quality of life in the community. More broadly, along with an increase in funding for research on the quality and outcome of treatment, such advances will provide program evaluators with a unique opportunity to help make a lasting improvement in our nationwide system of mental health care.

Appendix A

Ward Atmosphere Scale Scoring Key

This appendix contains the scoring key for the Ward Atmosphere Scale (WAS). The Real Form and Ideal Form are parallel; all items are scored in the same direction on both forms. An item listed as "true" (T) is scored one point if marked "true" by the individual completing the scale and an item listed as "false" (F) is scored one point if marked "false." The subscale score is the number of items answered in the scored direction.

The WAS and the third edition of the WAS Manual are published and are available for interested users (Moos, 1996b). The manual contains a copy of the WAS, normative and psychometric data, a review of practical and research applications of the scale, and standard score conversion tables to use in plotting WAS profiles. The user's guide to the Social Climate Scales (Moos, 1994b) discusses practical issues in scale administration and addresses some recurrent conceptual and methodological questions.

Involvement

Item Number	Scoring Direction	
1	T	Patients put a lot of energy into what they do around here.
11	T	This is a lively program.
21	T	The patients are proud of this program.
31	F	There is very little group spirit in this program.
41	F	Very few patients ever volunteer around here.
51	T	Patients are quite busy all of the time.
61	F	The program has very few social activities.
71	F	Very few things around here ever get people excited.
81	T	Discussions here are very interesting.
91	T	Patients often do things together on weekends.

Support

Item Number	Scoring Direction	
2	F	Doctors have very little time to encourage patients.
12	T	The staff know what the patients want.
22	T	Staff are interested in following up patients once they leave the program.
32	F	Nurses have very little time to encourage patients.
42	F	Doctors spend more time with some patients than with others.
52	T	The healthier patients here help take care of the less healthy ones.
62	F	Patients rarely help each other.
72	T	The staff help new patients get acquainted here.
82	F	Staff sometimes do not show up for their appointments with patients.
92	T	Staff go out of their way to help patients.

Spontaneity

Item Number	Scoring Direction	
3	F	Patients tend to hide their feelings from one another.
13	T	Patients say anything they want to the doctors.
23	F	It is hard to tell how patients are feeling here.
33	F	Patients are careful about what they say when staff are around.
43	T	Patients freely set up their own activities here.
53	F	When patients disagree with each other, they keep it to themselves.
63	T	It's okay to act crazy around here.
73	F	Patients tend to hide their feelings from the staff.
83	T	Patients are strongly encouraged to show their feelings.
93	(Filler item)	The program always stays just about the same.

Autonomy

Item Number	Scoring Direction	
4	T	The staff act on patients' suggestions.
14	F	Very few patients have any responsibility here.
24	T	Patients are expected to take leadership here.
34	T	Patients here are encouraged to be independent.
44	T	Patients can leave the unit whenever they want to.
54	T	Patients can wear whatever they want.
64	F	There is no patient government in this program.
74	T	Patients can leave the unit without saying where they are going.
84	F	Staff rarely give in to patients' pressure.
94	F	The staff discourage criticism.

Practical Orientation

Item Number	Scoring Direction	
5	T	New treatment approaches are often tried in this program.
15	F	There is very little emphasis on teaching patients solutions to practical problems.
25	T	Patients are strongly encouraged to plan for the future.
35	F	There is very little emphasis on what patients will be doing after they leave.
45	F	There is very little emphasis on making plans for getting out of this program.
55	T	This program emphasizes training for new kinds of jobs.
65	F	Most patients are more concerned with the past than with the future.
75	T	Patients are encouraged to learn new ways of doing things.
85	F	Staff care more about how patients feel than about their practical problems.
95	T	Patients must make specific plans before leaving the program.

Personal Problem Orientation

Item Number	Scoring Direction	
6	F	Patients hardly ever discuss their sex life.
16	T	Patients tell each other about their personal problems.
26	T	Personal problems are openly talked about.
36	T	Patients are expected to share their personal problems with each other.
46	F	Patients talk very little about their past.
56	F	The staff rarely ask patients personal questions.
66	T	Staff are mainly interested in learning about patients' feelings.
76	F	The patients rarely talk with each other about their personal problems.
86	T	Staff strongly encourage patients to talk about their past.
96	(Filler item)	It is hard to get a group together for card games or other activities.

Anger and Aggression

Item Number	Scoring Direction	
7	T	Patients often gripe.
17	T	Patients often criticize or joke about the staff.
27	F	Patients in this program rarely argue.
37	T	Staff sometimes argue openly with each other.
47	T	Patients sometimes play practical jokes on each other.
57	F	It's hard to get people to argue around here.
67	F	Staff here never start arguments.
77	T	In this program, staff think it is a healthy thing to argue.
87	F	Patients here rarely become angry.
97	(Filler item)	A lot of patients just seem to be passing time here.

Order and Organization

Item Number	Scoring Direction	
8	T	Patients' activities are carefully planned.
18	T	This is a very well organized program.
28	T	The staff make sure that the unit is always neat.
38	F	The unit sometimes gets very messy.
48	T	Most patients follow a regular schedule each day.
58	F	Many patients look messy.
68	F	Things are sometimes very disorganized around here.
78	T	The staff set an example for neatness and orderliness.
88	T	Patients are rarely kept waiting when they have appointments with staff.
98	F	The dayroom is often messy.

Program Clarity

Item Number	Scoring Direction	
9	T	The patients know when doctors will be on the unit.
19	F	Doctors do not explain what treatment is about to patients.
29	T	If a patient's medicine is changed, a nurse or doctor always explains why.
39	T	The patients clearly understand the program rules.
49	F	Patients never know when staff will ask to see them.
59	T	In this program, everyone knows who is in charge.
69	T	Patients who break the rules know what will happen to them.
79	F	People are always changing their minds here.
89	F	Patients never know when they will be transferred from this program.
99	T	Staff tell patients when they are getting better.

Staff Control

Item Number	Scoring Direction	
10	F	The staff very rarely punish patients by restricting them.
20	F	Patients may interrupt when a doctor is talking.
30	T	Patients who break the rules are punished for it.
40	T	Patients who argue with other patients will get into trouble with the staff.
50	F	Staff do not order the patients around.
60	T	Once a schedule is arranged for a patient, the patient must follow it.
70	F	Patients can call nursing staff by their first name.
80	T	Patients will be transferred from this program if they do not obey the rules.
90	T	It is not safe for patients to discuss their personal problems around here.
100	T	It is a good idea to let the doctors know that they are in charge.

Appendix B

Community-Oriented Programs
Environment Scale Scoring Key

This appendix contains the current scoring key for the Community-Oriented Programs Environment Scale (COPES). This scoring key incorporates six changes that were made in the original COPES items on the basis of new psychometric data (Moos, 1996a). The Real Form and Ideal Form are parallel; all items are scored in the same direction on both forms. An item listed as "true" (T) is scored one point if marked "true" by the individual completing the scale and an item listed as "false" (F) is scored one point is marked "false." The subscale score is the number of items answered in the scored direction.

The COPES and the third edition of the COPES Manual are published and are available for interested users (Moos, 1996a). The manual contains a copy of the COPES, normative and psychometric data, a review of practical and research applications of the scale, and standard score conversion tables to use in plotting COPES profiles. The user's guide to the Social Climate Scales (Moos, 1994b) discusses practical issues in scale administration and addresses some recurrent conceptual and methodological questions.

Involvement

Item Number	Scoring Direction	
1	T	Members put a lot of energy into what they do around here.
11	T	This is a lively program.
21	T	The members are proud of this program.
31	F	There is very little group spirit in this program.
41	F	Very few members ever volunteer around here.
51	F	A lot of members just seem to be passing time here.
61	F	This program has very few social activities.
71	T	Members are quite busy all of the time.
81	T	Discussions here are very interesting.
91	T	Members often do things together on weekends.

Support

Item Number	Scoring Direction	
2	T	The healthier members here help take care of the less healthy ones.
12	F	Staff have very little time to encourage members.
22	F	Members seldom help each other.
32	T	Staff are very interested in following up members once they leave the program.
42	T	Staff always compliment a member who does something well.
52	T	The staff know what the members want.
62	F	Staff sometimes do not show up for their appointments with members.
72	F	There is relatively little sharing among the members.
82	T	Members are given a great deal of individual attention here.
92	T	The staff go out of their way to help new members get acquainted here.

Spontaneity

Item Number	Scoring Direction	
3	F	Members tend to hide their feelings from one another.
13	T	Members say anything they want to the staff.
23	F	It is hard to tell how members are feeling here.
33	F	Members are careful about what they say when staff are around.
43	T	Members are strongly encouraged to express themselves freely here.
53	T	Members spontaneously set up their own activities here.
63	F	When members disagree with each other, they keep it to themselves.
73	T	Members can generally do whatever they feel like here.
83	F	Members tend to hide their feelings from the staff.
93	T	Members are strongly encouraged to express their feelings.

Autonomy

Item Number	Scoring Direction	
4	F	There is no membership government in this program.
14	T	Members have a say in making the rules.
24	T	Members are expected to take leadership here.
34	F	The staff discourage criticism.
44	T	Members can leave the program whenever they want to.
54	T	Members often take charge of activities.
64	T	The staff almost always act on members' suggestions.
74	F	Very few members have any responsibility here.
84	T	Members here are very strongly encouraged to be independent.
94	F	Members usually wait for staff to suggest an idea or activity.

Practical Orientation

Item Number	Scoring Direction	
5	T	This program emphasizes training for new kinds of jobs.
15	F	There is relatively little emphasis on teaching members solutions to practical problems.
25	T	Members are expected to make detailed, specific plans for the future.
35	F	There is relatively little discussion about exactly what members will be doing after they leave the program.
45	F	There is relatively little emphasis on making specific plans for leaving this program.
55	F	Most members are more concerned with the past than with the future.
65	T	Members here are expected to demonstrate continued concrete progress toward their goals.
75	T	Members are taught specific new skills in this program.
85	T	Staff strongly encourage members to do things in the community.
95	T	Members must make detailed plans before leaving the program.

Personal Problem Orientation

Item Number	Scoring Direction	
6	F	Members hardly ever discuss their sex life.
16	T	Personal problems are openly talked about.
26	F	The staff rarely ask members personal questions.
36	T	Members are expected to share their personal problems with each other.
46	F	Members talk relatively little about their past.
56	T	Members tell each other about their intimate personal problems.
66	T	Staff are mainly interested in learning about members' feelings.
76	F	The members seldom talk with each other about their personal problems.
86	F	Members are rarely encouraged to discuss their personal problems here.
96	T	Staff strongly encourage members to talk about their past.

Anger and Aggression

Item Number	Scoring Direction	
7	F	It is hard to get people to argue around here.
17	T	Members often criticize or joke about the staff.
27	F	Members here rarely argue.
37	T	Staff sometimes argue openly with each other.
47	T	Members sometimes play practical jokes on each other.
57	T	Staff encourage members to express their anger openly here.
67	F	Staff here never start arguments.
77	T	Members often gripe.
87	T	Staff here think it is a healthy thing to argue.
97	F	Members here rarely become angry.

Order and Organization

Item Number	Scoring Direction	
8	T	Members' activities are carefully planned.
18	T	This is a very well organized program.
28	T	The staff make sure that this place is always neat.
38	F	This place usually looks a little messy.
48	T	Members here follow a regular schedule every day.
58	F	Some members look messy.
68	F	Things are sometimes very disorganized around here.
78	F	The dayroom or living room is often untidy.
88	T	Members are rarely kept waiting when they have appointments with staff.
98	T	The staff strongly encourage members to be neat and orderly.

Clarity

Item Number	Scoring Direction	
9	T	Members who break the rules, know what the consequences will be.
19	T	If a member's program is changed, staff always explain why.
29	F	Staff rarely give members a detailed explanation of what the program is about.
39	T	The members clearly understand the program rules.
49	F	Members never know when staff will ask to see them.
59	T	The members always know when the staff will be around.
69	T	Everyone knows who is in charge of this program.
79	F	People are always changing their minds here.
89	F	Members never know when they will be considered ready to leave the program.
99	F	There are often changes in the rules here.

Staff Control

Item Number	Scoring Direction	
10	T	Once a schedule is arranged for a member, the member must follow it.
20	F	The staff very rarely punish members by taking away their privileges.
30	T	Members who break the rules are punished for it.
40	T	Members who fight with other members will get into trouble with the staff.
50	F	Staff do not order the members around.
60	T	It is important to carefully follow the program rules here.
70	F	Members can wear whatever they want.
80	F	Members may interrupt staff when they are talking.
90	T	Members will be transferred or discharged from this program if they do not obey the rules.
100	F	Members can refuse to participate in planned program activities.

References

Alden, L. (1978a). Factor analysis of the word atmosphere scale. *Journal of Consulting and Clinical Psychology* 46: 175–76.

———. (1978b). Treatment environment and patient improvement. *Journal of Nervous and Mental Disease* 166: 327–34.

Alexy, W. (1981–82). Perceptions of ward atmosphere on an oncology unit. *International Journal of Psychiatry in Medicine* 11: 331–40.

Allen, C. I., Gillespie, C. R., and Hall, J. N. (1989). A comparison of practices, attitudes and interactions in two established units for people with a psychiatric disability. *Psychological Medicine* 19: 459–67.

Allen, K. (1993). Current morale issues that impede the caregiving process of substance abuse/addictions nurses. *Issues in Mental Health Nursing* 14: 293–305.

Amaral, P., Nehemkis, A., and Fox, L. (1981). Staff support group on a cancer ward: A pilot project. *Death Education* 5: 267–78.

Appelbaum, A. H., and Munich, R. L. (1986). Reinventing moral treatment: The effects upon patients and staff members of a program of psychosocial rehabilitation. *The Psychiatric Hospital* 17: 11–19.

Apte, R. (1968). *Halfway Houses*. London: Bell and Sons.

Arrington, B., and Haddock, C. C. (1990). Who really profits from not-for-profits? *Health Services Research* 25: 291–304.

Azrin, N. (1976). Improvements in the community reinforcement approach to alcoholism. *Behavior Research and Therapy* 14: 339–48.

Azrin, N., Sisson, R., Meyers, R., and Godley, M. (1982). Alcoholism treatment by disulfiram and community reinforcement therapy. *Journal of Behavioral Therapy and Experimental Psychiatry* 13: 105–12.

Baird, J. W. (1987). Locus-of-control, self-reported depression and perception of ward atmosphere in psychiatric patients (Doctoral dissertation, University of Pittsburgh, 1985). *Dissertation Abstracts International* 47: 2505.

Bakos, M., Bozic, R., Chapin, D., and Neuman, S. (1980). Effects of environmental changes on elderly residents' behavior. *Hospital and Community Psychiatry* 31: 677–82.

Baldwin, S. (1985). Effects of furniture rearrangement on the atmosphere of wards in a maximum security hospital. *Hospital and Community Psychiatry* 36: 525–28.

271

272   **Evaluating Treatment Environments**

Bale, R., Zarcone, V., Van Stone, W., Kuldau, J., Engelsing, T., and Elashoff, R. (1984). Three therapeutic communities: Process and outcome in a prospective controlled study of narcotic addiction treatment. *Archives of General Psychiatry* 41: 185–91.

Barker, S. B., and Barker, R. T. (1994). Managing change in an interdisciplinary inpatient unit: An action research approach. *Journal of Mental Health Administration* 21: 80–91.

Bausell, R. B., Rinkus, A., and Watson, D. (1979). The relationship between treatment modality, demographic characteristics, and staff perceptions concerning their jobs in 26 Philadelphia drug treatment centers. *International Journal of the Addictions* 14: 99–109.

Beard, J. H., Propst, R. N., and Malamud, T. J. (1982). The fountain house model of psychiatric rehabilitation. *Psychosocial Rehabilitation Journal* 5: 47–53.

Belknap, I. (1956). *Human Problems of a State Mental Hospital.* New York: McGraw Hill.

Bell, M. (1983). The perceived social environment of a therapeutic community for drug abusers. *International Journal of Therapeutic Communities* 4: 262–70.

———. (1985). Three therapeutic communities for drug abusers: Differences in treatment environments. *Journal of the Addictions* 20: 1523–31.

Bell, M., and Ryan, E. (1984). Integrating psychosocial rehabilitation into the hospital psychiatric service. *Hospital and Community Psychiatry* 35: 1017–23.

———. (1985). Where can therapeutic community ideals be realized? An examination of biologic, psychoanalytic and rehabilitation treatment environments. *Hospital and Community Psychiatry* 36: 1286–91.

Bernstein, E., Heim, E., and Ballinari, P. (1983). Milieu-interaction schizophrener. *Nervenarzt* 54: 590–97.

Blacker, E., and Kantor, D. (1960). Halfway houses for problem drinkers. *Federal Probation* 24: 18–23.

Bliss, F., Moos, R., and Bromet, E. (1976). Monitoring change in a community-oriented treatment program. *Journal of Community Psychology* 4: 315–26.

Blotcky, M. J., Dimperio, T. L., and Gossett, J. T. (1984). Follow-up of children treated in psychiatric hospitals: A review of studies. *The American Journal of Psychiatry* 141: 1499–1507.

Bocker, F. M. (1989). Zufriedenheit psychisch kranker mit der psychiatrischen klinikbehandlung. *Psycho: Psychiatrie, Neurologie und Psychotherapie fur Klinik und Praxis* 15: 608–20.

Bootzin, R. R., Shadish, W. R., and McSweeny, A. J. (1989). Longitudinal outcomes of nursing home care for severely mentally ill patients. *Journal of Social Issues* 45: 31–48.

Boyd, M. A., Luetje, V., and Eckert, A. (1992). Creating organizational change in an inpatient long-term care facility. *Psychosocial Rehabilitation Journal* 15: 47–54.

Boydell, K. M., and Everett, B. (1992). What makes a house a home? An evaluation of a supported housing project for individuals with long-term psychiatric backgrounds. *Canadian Journal of Community Mental Health* 10: 109–23.

Brennan, P., and Moos, R. (1990). Physical design, social climate, and staff turnover in skilled nursing facilities. *Journal of Long-Term Care Administration* 18: 22–27.

Brown, P. (1985). *The transfer of care: Psychiatric deinstitutionalization and its aftermath.* London: Routledge and Kegan Paul.

Burda, P. C., Starkey, T. W., Dominguez, F., and Fernandez, E. (1991). A biopsychosocial approach to the chronic psychiatric patient. *VA Practitioner* 8: 55–60.

Burti, L., Glick, I. D., and Tansella, M. (1990). Measuring the treatment environment of a psychiatric ward and a community mental health center after the Italian reform. *Community Mental Health Journal* 26: 193–204.

Cahn, S. (1969). Alcoholism halfway houses: Relationships to other programs and facilities. *Social Work* 14: 50–60.

Caplan, C. A. (1993). Nursing staff and patient perceptions of the ward atmosphere in a maximum security forensic hospital. *Archives of Psychiatric Nursing* 7: 23–29.

Carroll, R. S., Miller, A., Ross, B., and Simpson, G. M. (1980). Research as an impetus to improved treatment. *Archives of General Psychiatry* 37: 377–80.

Caudill, W. (1958). *The psychiatric hospital as a small society*. Cambridge, Mass.: Harvard University Press.

Christenfeld, R., Wagner, J., Pastva, G., and Acrish, W. P. (1989). How physical settings affect chronic mental patients. *Psychiatric Quarterly* 60: 253–64.

Cohen, S., and Khan, A. (1990). Antipsychotic effect of milieu in the acute treatment of schizophrenia. *General Hospital Psychiatry* 12: 248–51.

Collins, J., Ellsworth, R., Casey, N., Hickey, R., and Hyer, L. (1984). Treatment characteristics of effective psychiatric programs. *Hospital and Community Psychiatry* 35: 601–05.

Collins, J., Ellsworth, R., Casey, N., Hyer, L., Hickey, R., Schoonover, R., Twemlow, S., and Nesselroade, J. (1985). Treatment characteristics of psychiatric programs that correlate with patient community adjustment. *Journal of Clinical Psychology* 41: 299–308.

Comstock, B. S., Kamiliar, S. M., Thornby, J. I., Ramirez, J. V., and Kaplan, H. B. (1985). Crisis treatment in a day hospital: Impact on medical care-seeking. *Psychiatric Clinics of North America* 8: 483–500.

Cook, C. (1988). The Minnesota Model in the management of drug and alcohol dependency: Miracle, method or myth? Part I. The philosophy and the programme. *British Journal of Addiction* 83: 625–34.

Cooper, L. (1973). Staff attitudes about ideal wards before and after program change. *Journal of Community Psychology* 1: 82–83.

Corey, L. J., Wallace, M. A., Harris, S. H., and Casey, D. (1986). A before and after look at how refurbishing affects staff and patient perceptions of the psycho-social treatment environment. *Journal of Psychosocial Nursing* 24: 10–16.

Coulton, C. J., Holland, T. E., and Fitch, V. (1984a). Person-environment congruence and psychiatric patient outcome in community care homes. *Administration in Mental Health* 12: 71–88.

———. (1984b). Person-environment congruence as a predictor of early rehospitalization from community care homes. *Psychosocial Rehabilitation Journal* 8: 24–37.

Coyne, L., Smith, M. J., Deering, C. D., Grame, C. Langworthy, D. E., Rooks, T. E., Taylor, M. W., and Spohn, H. E. (1990). Outcome at discharge for patients in an ongoing follow-up study of hospital treatment. *Hospital and Community Psychiatry* 41: 657–62.

Crisler, J., and Settles, R. (1979). An integrated rehabilitation team effort in providing services for multiple disability clients. *Journal of Rehabilitation* 45: 34–38.

Cronkite, R., and Moos, R. (1978). Evaluating alcoholism treatment programs: An integrated approach. *Journal of Consulting and Clinical Psychology* 46: 1105–19.

————. (1984). Sex and marital status in relation to the treatment and outcome of alcoholic patients. *Sex Roles* 11: 93–112.

Cruser, D. A. (1995). Evaluating program design in the state hospital setting. *Journal of Mental Health Administration* 22: 49–57.

Culhane, D. P., and Hadley, T. R. (1992). The discriminating characteristics of for-profit versus not-for-profit freestanding psychiatric inpatient facilities. *Health Services Research* 27: 178–94.

Curtiss, S. (1976). The compatibility of humanistic and behavioristic approaches in a state mental hospital. In A. Wandersman, P. Poppen, and D. Ricks (Eds.), *Humanism and behaviorism: Dialogue and growth* (235–51). New York: Pergamon Press.

Dauwalder, J., Chabloz, D., and Chappuis, J. (1978). L'echelle de l'atmosphere dans les services psychiatriques (A scale to measure the atmosphere of psychiatric programs). *Social Psychiatry* 13: 175–86.

Davis, R. C. (1985). The relationship between residential program characteristics and patients' integration into the community and satisfaction with their living environment (Doctoral dissertation, Michigan State University, 1984). *Dissertation Abstracts International* 46: 637B.

Deering, C. D., Coyne, L., Grame, C. J., Smith, M. J., Rooks, T. E., Taylor, M. W., Langworthy, D. E., and Spohn, H. E. (1991). Effects of extended hospitalization: A one-year follow-up study. *Bulletin of the Menninger Clinic* 55: 444–53.

DeLeon, G. (1973). The Phoenix House therapeutic community: Changes in psychopathological signs. *Archives of General Psychiatry* 28: 131–35.

De-Nour, A. K. (1983). Staff-patient interaction. In N. Levy (Ed.), *Psychonephrology: Psychological problems in kidney failure and their treatment* (Vol. 2, 31–41). New York: Plenum Press.

Denny, N., Costello, R., and Cochran, M. (1984). Factor implied scales of ward atmosphere. *Evaluation and the Health Professions* 7: 181–92.

Devlin, A. S. (1992). Psychiatric ward renovation: Staff perception and patient behavior. *Environment and Behavior* 24: 66–84.

Dickens, C. (1842). *American notes for general circulation* (Vol. 1). London: Chapman.

Doherty, E. (1976). Length of hospitalization on a short-term therapeutic community: A multivariate study by sex across time. *Archives of General Psychiatry* 33: 87–92.

Doniger, J., Rothwell, N., and Cohen, R. (1963). Case study of a halfway house. *Mental Hospitals* 14: 191–99.

Dorr, D., Honea, S., and Pozner, R. (1980). Ward atmosphere and psychiatric nurses' job satisfaction. *American Journal of Community Psychology* 8: 455–61.

Downs, M. W., and Fox, J. C. (1993). Social environments of adult homes. *Community Mental Health Journal* 29: 15–23.

Drake, R. E., Mueser, K. T., Clark, R. E., and Wallach, M. A. (1996). The course, treatment, and outcome of substance disorder in persons with severe mental illness. *American Journal of Orthopsychiatry* 66: 42–51.

Ejsing, L. O. (1980). Ward Atmosphere scale anvendt i arbejdet med at mindske afstanden mellem idealer og oplevede realiteter i et terapeutisk samfund. *Nordisk Psykiatrisk Tidsskrift* 34: 658–71.

Ellsworth, R., Casey, N., Hickey, R., Twemlow, S., Collins, J., Schoonover, R., Hyer, L., and Nesselroade, J. (1979). Some characteristics of effective psychiatric treatment programs. *Journal of Consulting and Clinical Psychology* 47: 799–817.

Ellsworth, R., Maroney, R., Klett, W., Gordon, H., and Gunn, R. (1971). Milieu characteristics of successful psychiatric treatment programs. *American Journal of Orthopsychiatry* 41: 427–41.

Elzinga, R. H., and Barlow, J. (1991). Patient satisfaction among the residential population of a psychiatric hospital. *The International Journal of Social Psychiatry* 37: 24–34.

Eriksen, L. (1987). Ward atmosphere changes during restructuring of an alcoholism treatment center: A quasi-experimental study. *Addictive Behaviors* 12: 33–42.

Erikson, E. (1950). *Childhood and society.* New York: Norton.

Fairchild, H., and Wright, C. (1984). A social-ecological assessment and feedback intervention of an adolescent treatment agency. *Adolescence* 19: 263–75.

Fairweather, G. (Ed.). (1964). *Social psychology in treating mental illness: An experimental approach.* New York: Wiley.

Fairweather, G., Sanders, D., Cressler, D., and Maynard, H. (1969). *Community life for the mentally ill: An alternative to institutional care.* Chicago: Aldine.

Farndale, J. (1961). *The day hospital movement in Great Britain.* London: Pergamon Press.

Feist, J. R., Slowiak, C. A., and Colligan, R. C. (1985). Beyond good intentions: Applying scientific methods to the art of milieu therapy. *Residential Group Care and Treatment* 3: 13–32.

Finnema, E. J., Dassen, T., and Halfens, R. (1994). Aggression in psychiatry: A qualitative study focusing on the characterization and perception of patient aggression by nurses working on psychiatric wards. *Journal of Advanced Nursing* 19: 1088–95.

Finney, J. (1995). Enhancing substance abuse treatment evaluations: Examining mediators and moderators of treatment effects. *Journal of Substance Abuse* 7: 135–50.

Finney, J. Hahn, A., and Moos, R. (1996). The effectiveness of inpatient and outpatient treatment for alcohol abuse: The need to focus on mediators and moderators of setting effects. *Addiction* 91.

Finney, J., and Monahan, S. (1996). The cost effectiveness of treatment for alcoholism: A second approximation. *Journal of Studies on Alcohol* 57.

Finney, J., and Moos, R. (1992). The long-term course of treated alcoholism: II. Predictors and correlates of 10-year functioning and mortality. *Journal of Studies on Alcohol* 53: 142–53.

Fischer, J. (1977). Alcoholic patients' perception of treatment milieu using modified versions of the Ward Atmosphere Scale (WAS) and Community-Oriented Programs Environment Scale (COPES). *British Journal of Addiction* 72: 213–16.

———. (1979). The relationship between alcoholic patients' milieu perception and measures of their drinking during a brief follow-up period. *International Journal of the Addictions* 14: 1151–56.

Flaherty, J., Naidu, J., Lawton, R., and Pathak, D. (1981). Racial differences in perception of ward atmosphere. *American Journal of Psychiatry* 138: 815–17.

Flaherty, J., Naidu, J., Lawton, R., and Verinis, S. (1980). The effects of geographic relocations on a general hospital's psychiatric units. *Hospital and Community Psychiatry* 31: 819–21.

Flannery, R. B., Hanson, M. A., and Penk, W. E. (1994). Risk factors for psychiatric inpatient assaults on staff. *Journal of Mental Health Administration* 21: 24–31.

Friedman, A. S., and Glickman, N. W. (1986). Program characteristics for successful treatment of adolescent drug abuse. *Journal of Nervous and Mental Diseases, 174,* 669-679.

———. (1987). Residential program characteristics for completion of treatment by adolescent drug abusers. *Journal of Nervous and Mental Diseases* 175: 419–24.

Friedman, A. S., Glickman, N. W., and Kovach, J. A. (1986a). Comparisons of perceptions of the environments of adolescent drug treatment residential and outpatient programs by staff versus clients and by sex of staff and clients. *American Journal of Drug and Alcohol Abuse* 12: 31–52.

———. (1986b). The relationship of drug program environmental variables to treatment outcome. *American Journal of Drug and Alcohol Abuse* 12: 53–69.

Friedman, S. (1982). Consultation for self-evaluation: Social climate assessment as a catalyst for programmatic change in mental health treatment environments. In A. Jeger and R. Slotnick (Eds.), *Community mental health and behavioral ecology: A handbook of theory, research and practice* (187–96). New York: Plenum Press.

Friedman, S., Jeger, A., and Slotnick, R. (1980). Psychosocial climate of a psychiatric ward: Differential perceptions of nursing personnel and other professionals. *American Journal of Community Psychology* 8: 613–15.

———. (1982). Social ecological assessment of mental health treatment environments: Towards self-evaluation. *Psychological Reports* 50: 631–38.

Friis, S. (1980). Idealposten-Ideell for hvem? *Scandinavian Journal of Psychiatry* 34: 120–28.

———. (1981a). From enthusiasm to resignation in a therapeutic community: A process evaluation of a mental hospital ward with the Ward Atmosphere Scale (WAS). *Journal of the Oslo City Hospitals* 31: 51–54.

———. (1981b). Hva slags postatmosfaere er terapeutisk for psykotiske og for ikkepsykotiske pasienter? *Journal of the Norwegian Medical Association* 101: 848–52.

———. (1986a). Characteristics of a good ward atmosphere. *Acta Psychiatrica Scandinavica* 74: 469–73.

———. (1986b). Factors influencing the ward atmosphere. *Acta Psychiatrica Scandinavica* 73: 600–06.

———. (1991). What is the importance of the milieu for the occurrence of violence in psychiatric wards? *Nordic Journal of Psychiatry* 45 (suppl. 25): 21–26.

Friis, S., Karterud, S., Kleppe, H., Lorentzen, S., Lystrup, S., and Vaglum, P. (1982). Reconsidering some limiting factors of therapeutic communities a summary of six norwegian studies. In M. Pines and L. Rafaelsen (Eds.), *The individual and the group: Boundaries and interrelations.* Volume I: Theory (573–81). New York: Plenum.

Garety, P. A., and Morris, I. (1984). A new unit for long-stay psychiatric patients: Organization, attitudes and quality of care. *Psychological Medicine* 14: 183–92.

Geller, J. L. (1991). Anyplace but the state hospital: Examining assumptions about the benefits of admission diversion. *Hospital and Community Psychiatry* 42: 145–52.

Glasscote, R., Glassman, S., Jepson, W., and Kraft, A. (1969). *Partial hospitalization for the mentally ill: A study of programs and problems.* Washington, D.C.: American Psychiatric Association.

Glasscote, R., Gudeman, J., and Elpers, R. (1971). *Halfway houses for the mentally ill.* Washington, D.C.: Joint Information Service of the American Psychiatric Association.

Glick, I., and Hargreaves, W. (1979). *Psychiatric hospital treatment for the 1980s: A controlled study of short versus long hospitalization.* Lexington, Mass.: D. C. Heath.

Goffman, E. (1961). *Asylums: Essays on the social situation of mental patients and other inmates.* Garden City, N.Y.: Doubleday.

Goldmeier, J., and Silver, S. B. (1988). Women staff members and ward atmospheres in a forensic hospital. *International Journal of Offender Therapy and Comparative Criminology* 32: 257–65.

Goldstein, J. M., Cohen, P., Lewis, S. A., and Struening, E. L. (1988). Community treatment environments: Patient vs. staff evaluations. *Journal of Nervous and Mental Disease* 176: 227—33.

Grant, R., and Saslow, G. (1971). Maximizing responsible decisionmaking, or how do we get out of here? In G. Abroms and N. Greenfield (Eds.), *The new hospital psychiatry* (27–55). New York: Academic Press.

Greenberg, E., Obitz, F., and Kaye, D. (1978). Relationships among control orientation, the FIRO-B and the Ward Atmosphere Scale in hospitalized men alcoholics. *Journal of Studies on Alcohol* 39: 68–76.

Greenberg, J. (1964). *I never promised you a rose garden*. New York: Holt, Rinehart and Winston.

Gripp, R., and Magaro, P. (1971). A token economy program evaluation with untreated control ward comparisons. *Behavior Research and Therapy* 9: 137–39.

Grob, G. (1966). *The state and the mentally ill: A history of Worcester State Hospital in Massachusetts, 1830–1920*. Chapel Hill, N.C.: University of North Carolina Press.

Grob, G. (1980). Institutional origins and early transformation: 1830–1855. In J. P. Morrissey, H. H. Goldman, and L. V. Klerman, (Eds.), *The enduring asylum: Cycles of institutional reform at Worcester State Hospital* (19–44). New York: Grune and Stratton.

Gunderson, J. G. (1983). If and when milieu therapy is therapeutic for schizophrenics. In J. G. Gunderson, O. A. Will, and L. R. Mosher (Eds.), *Principles and Practice of Milieu Therapy* (57–66). New York: Aronson.

Halford, W. K., and Hayes, R. (1991). Psychological rehabilitation of chronic schizophrenic patients: Recent findings on social skills training and family psychoeducation. *Clinical Psychology Review* 11: 23–44.

Hall, S., Bass, A., Hargreaves, W., and Loeb, P. (1979). Contingency management and information feedback in outpatient heroin detoxification. *Behavior Therapy* 10: 443—51.

Hansson, L. (1989). Patient satisfaction with in-hospital psychiatric care: A study of a 1-year population of patients hospitalized in a sectorized care organization. *European Archives of Psychiatry and Neurological Sciences* 239: 93–100.

Hansson, L., and Berglund, M. (1987). Factors influencing treatment outcome and patient satisfaction in a short-term psychiatric ward: A path analysis study of the importance of patient involvement in treatment planning. *European Archives of Psychiatry and Neurological Sciences* 236: 269–75.

Hansson, L., Bjorkman, T., and Berglund, I. (1993). What is important in psychiatric inpatient care? Quality of care from the patient's perspective. *Quality Assurance in Health Care* 5: 41–47.

Harris, R., Linn, M., and Pratt, T. (1980). A comparison of dropouts and disciplinary discharges from a therapeutic community. *International Journal of the Addictions* 15: 749–56.

Hartmann, H. (1951). Ego psychology and the problems of adaptation. In D. Rapaport (Ed.), *Organization and pathology of thought* (361–96). New York: Columbia University Press.

Hattie, J. A., Sharpley, C. F., and Rogers, H. J. (1984). Comparative effectiveness of paraprofessional and professional helpers. *Psychological Bulletin* 95: 534–41.

278   Evaluating Treatment Environments

Hellman, I., Greene, L., Morrison, T., and Abramowitz, S. (1985). Organizational size and perception in a residential treatment program. *American Journal of Community Psychology* 13: 99–109.

Herrera, J. M., and Lawson, W. B. (1987). Effects of consultation on the ward atmosphere in a state psychiatric hospital. *Psychological Reports* 60: 423–28.

Hills, A. A. (1987). Adjustment to relocation of long-stay patients with a psychiatric hospital setting. *Psychological Reports* 60: 123–28.

Holland, J. (1985). *Making vocational choices: A theory of careers.* Englewood Cliffs, N.J.: Prentice Hall.

Houts, P., and Moos, R. (1969). The development of a Ward Initiative Scale for patients. *Journal of Clinical Psychology* 25: 319–22.

Ingstad, J., and Gotestam, K. G. (1979). A three level approach to the evaluation of a therapeutic community system. *World Conference of Therapeutic Communities* 3: 351–63.

Jackson, J. (1969). Factors of the treatment environment. *Archives of General Psychiatry* 21: 39–45.

James, I., Milne, D. L., and Firth, H. (1990). A systematic comparison of feedback and staff discussion in changing the ward atmosphere. *Journal of Advanced Nursing* 15: 329–36.

Jansen, E. (Ed.) (1980). *The Therapeutic Community.* London: Croom Helm.

Johnson, S. (1981). Staff cohesion in residential treatment. *Journal of Youth and Adolescence* 10: 221–32.

Jones, M. (1953). *The therapeutic community: A new treatment method in psychiatry.* New York: Basic Books.

Kahn, E. M., Storke, I. T., and Schaeffer, J. (1992). Inpatient group processes parallel unit dynamics. *International Journal of Group Psychotherapy* 42: 407–19.

Kahn, E. M., and White, E. M. (1989). Adapting milieu approaches to acute inpatient care for schizophrenic patients. *Hospital and Community Psychiatry* 40: 609–14.

Kanter, R. M. (1972). *Commitment and community.* Cambridge, Mass.: Harvard University Press.

Kellam, S., Sheppard, G., Goldberg, A., Schooler, N., Berman, A., and Shmelzer, J. (1967). Ward atmosphere and outcome of treatment of acute schizophrenia. *Journal of Psychiatric Research* 5: 145–63.

Keller, O., and Alper, B. (1970). *Halfway houses: Community-centered correction and treatment.* Lexington, Mass.: Heath-Lexington.

Kelly, G. R. (1983). Minimizing the adverse effects of mass relocation among chronic psychiatric inpatients. *Hospital and Community Psychiatry* 34: 150–57.

Kennard, D. (1983). *An introduction to therapeutic communities.* London: Routledge and Kegan Paul.

Kesey, K. (1962). *One flew over the cuckoo's nest.* New York: Viking.

Keso, L., and Salaspuro, M. (1990). Inpatient treatment of employed alcoholics: A randomized clinical trial of Hazelden-type and traditional treatment. *Alcoholism: Clinical and Experimental Research* 14: 584–89.

Kessler, R. C., Nelson, C. B., McGonagle, K. A., Edlund, M. J., Frank, R. G., and Leaf, P. J. (1996). The epidemology of co-occurring addictive and mental disorders: Implications for prevention and service utilization. *American Journal of Orthopsychiatry* 66: 17–31.

King, R., and Raynes, N. (1968). An operational measure of inmate management in residential institutions. *Social Science and Medicine* 2: 41–43.

Kish, G. (1971). Evaluation of ward atmosphere. *Hospital and Community Psychiatry* 22: 159–61.

Kish, G., Solberg, K., and Uecker, A. (1971a). Locus of control as a factor influencing patients' perceptions of ward atmosphere. *Journal of Clinical Psychology* 27: 287–89.

———. (1971b). The relation of staff opinions about mental illness to ward atmosphere and perceived staff roles. *Journal of Clinical Psychology* 27: 284–87.

Klass, D., Growe, G., and Strizich, M. (1977). Ward treatment milieu and post-hospital functioning. *Archives of General Psychiatry* 34: 1047–52.

Klein, R., Pillsbury, J., Bushey, M., and Snell, S. (1972). Psychiatric staff: Uniforms or street clothes? *Archives of General Psychiatry* 26: 19–22.

Kobos, J., Redmond, F., and Sterling, J. (1982). Measuring ward milieu and the impact of staff turnover on a psychiatry unit. *Psychological Reports* 50: 879–85.

Koran, L., Moos, R., Moos, B., and Zasslow, M. (1983). Changing hospital work environments: An example of a burn unit. *General Hospital Psychiatry* 5: 7–13.

Kyrouz, E., and Humphreys, K. (1996). *Do health care work places affect the treatment environment?* Palo Alto, Calif.: Department of Veterans Affairs, Center for Health Care Evaluation.

Lacoursiere, R., and Bradshaw, S. (1983). Problems in a treatment program for substance misuse: The process of reorganizing into assessment teams and modules. *Journal of Studies on Alcohol* 44: 647–64.

Lamb, R. (1994). A century and a half of psychiatric rehabilitation in the United States. *Hospital and Community Psychiatry* 45: 1015–20.

Lamb, R., and Goertzel, V. (1972). High expectations of long-term ex-state hospital patients. *American Journal of Psychiatry* 129: 131–35.

Landy, D. (1960). Rutland corner house: Case study of a halfway house. *Journal of Social Issues* 16: 27–32.

Langenbucher, J. (1994). Offsets are not add-ons: The place of addictions treatment in American health care reform. *Journal of Substance Abuse* 6: 117–22.

Lanza, M. L., Kayne, H. L., Hicks, C., and Milner, J. (1994). Environmental characteristics related to patient assault. *Issues in Mental Health Nursing* 15: 319–35.

Lavender, A. (1987). Improving the quality of care on psychiatric hospital rehabilitation wards: A controlled evaluation. *British Journal of Psychiatry* 150: 476–81.

Lawton, M. P. (1989). Behavior-relevant ecological factors. In K. W. Schaie and C. Schoder (Eds.), *Social structure and aging: Psychological processes* (57–78). Hillsdale, N.J.: Erlbaum.

Leda, C., Rosenheck, R., and Fontana, A. (1991). Impact of staffing levels on transitional residential treatment programs for homeless veterans. *Psychosocial Rehabilitation Journal* 15: 55–67.

Leda, C., Rosenheck, R., Medak, S., and Olson, R. (1989). *Healing communities: The second progress report on the Department of Veterans Affairs Domiciliary Care for Homeless Veterans Program.* West Haven, Conn.: Northeast Program Evaluation Center, Department of Veterans Affairs Medical Center.

———. (1990). Advances on the home front: Domiciliary care for homeless veterans. *VA Practitioner* 7: 91–92, 97–98, 101–03.

Leff, J., Dayson, D., Gooch, C., Thornicroft, G., and Wills, W. (1996). Quality of life of long-stay patients discharged from two psychiatric institutions. *Psychiatric Services* 47: 62–67.

Lehman, A. F., and Ritzler, B. (1976). The therapeutic community inpatient ward: Does it really work? *Comprehensive Psychiatry* 17: 755–61.

Lehman, A. F., Slaughter, J. G., and Myers, C. P. (1991). Quality of life in alternative residential settings. *Psychiatric Quarterly* 62: 35–49.

Lehman, A. F., Strauss, J. S., Ritzler, B. A., Kokes, R. F., Harder, D. W., and Gift, T. E. (1982). First admission psychiatric ward milieu: Treatment process and outcome. *Archives of General Psychiatry* 39: 1293–98.

Leiberich, P., Erlangen, von Cranach, M., Kaufbeuren, Hippius, H., and Munchen (1993). Verbesserung des stationsklimas auf akutpsychiatrischen stationen. *Psychiatrische Praxis* 20: 136–40.

Lemke, S., and Moos, R. (1987). Measuring the social climate of congregate residences for older people: Sheltered Care Environment Scale. *Psychology and Aging* 2: 20—29.

Leviege, V. (1970). Group relations: Group therapy with mentally ill offenders. *Corrective Psychiatry and Journal of Social Therapy* 16: 15–25.

Liberman, R. P. (1988). *Psychiatric Rehabilitation of Chronic Mental Patients*. Washington, D.C.: American Psychiatric Press, Inc.

Lieberman, P. B., Von Rehn, S., Dickie, E., Elliott, B., and Egerter, E. (1992). Therapeutic effects of brief hospitalization: The role of a therapeutic alliance. *The Journal of Psychotherapy Practice and Research* 1: 56–63.

Lindsay, J. S. B. (1986). The general hospital and the therapeutic community in North Queensland. *International Journal of Therapeutic Communities* 7: 129–38.

Linn, M. (1978). Attrition of older alcoholics from treatment. *Addictive Diseases* 3: 437–47.

Linn, M., Gurel, L., Williford, W. O., Overall, J., Gurland, B., Laughlin, P., and Barchiesi, A. (1985). Nursing home care as an alternative to psychiatric hospitalization. *Archives of General Psychiatry* 42: 544–51.

Linn, M., Shane, R., Webb, N., and Pratt, T. (1979). Cultural factors and attrition in drug abuse treatment. *International Journal of the Addictions* 14: 259–80.

Linn, M., and Stein, S. (1989). Nursing homes as community mental health facilities. In D. A. Rochefort (Ed.), *Handbook on mental health policy in the United States* (267–92). Westport, Conn.: Greenwood.

Linton, R. (1945). *The cultural background of personality*. New York: Century.

Lipsey, M., and Wilson, D. B. (1993). The efficacy of psychological, educational, and behavioral treatment: Confirmation from meta-analysis. *American Psychologist* 48: 1181–1209.

Long, C. G., Blackwell, C. C., and Midgley, M. (1990). An evaluation of two systems of in-patient care in a general hospital psychiatric unit II: Measures of staff and patient performance. *Journal of Advanced Nursing* 15: 1436–42.

———. (1992). An evaluation of two systems of in-patient care in a general hospital psychiatric unit I: Staff and patient perceptions and attitudes. *Journal of Advanced Nursing* 17: 64–71.

Luft, L., and Fakhouri, J. (1979). A model for a comparative cost-effectiveness evaluation of two mental health partial care programs. *Evaluation and Program Planning* 2: 33–40.

MacDonald, L., Sibbald, B., and Hoare, C. (1988). Measuring patient satisfaction with life in a long-stay psychiatric hospital. *The International Journal of Social Psychiatry* 34: 292–304.

Main, S., McBride, A. B., and Austin, J. K. (1991). Patient and staff perceptions of a psychiatric ward environment. *Issues in Mental Health Nursing* 12: 149–57.

Makkai, T., and McAllister, I. (1992). Measuring social indicators in opinion surveys: A method to improve accuracy on sensitive questions. *Social Indicators Research* 27: 169–86.

Manderscheid, R., Koenig, G., and Silbergeld, S. (1978). Psychosocial factors for classroom, group, and ward. *Psychological Reports* 43: 555– 61.

Mann, T. (1952). *The magic mountain*. New York: Random House.

Manning, N. (1989). *The therapeutic community movement: Charisma and routinization*. London: Routledge.

Marone, J., and Desiderato, O. (1982). Effects of locus of control on perceived hospital environment. *Journal of Clinical Psychology* 38: 555–61.

Mattson, M. E., Allen, J. P., Longabaugh, R., Nickless, C. J., Connors, G. J., and Kadden, R. M. (1994). A chronological review of empirical studies matching alcoholic clients to treatment. *Journal of Study of Alcohol* 12: 164–29.

McAllister, I., and Makkai, T. (1991). Correcting for the underreporting of drug use in opinion surveys. *The International Journal of the Addictions* 26: 945–61.

McFarlane, W. J. G., Bowman, R. G., and MacInnes, M. (1980). Patient access to hospital records: A pilot project. *Canadian Journal of Psychiatry* 25: 497–502.

McGee, M., and Woods, D. (1978). Use of Moos' Ward Atmosphere Scale in a residential setting for mentally retarded adolescents. *Psychological Reports* 43: 580–82.

McGlashan, T. H. (1984). The Chestnut Lodge follow-up study: II. Long-term outcome of schizophrenia and the affective disorders. *Archives of General Psychiatry* 41: 586–601.

———. (1986). The Chestnut Lodge follow-up study: III. Long-term outcome of borderline personalities. *Archives of General Psychiatry* 43: 20–30.

McKenna, H. (1993). The effects of nursing models on quality of care. *Nursing Times* 89: 43–46.

McLellan, A. T., Alterman, A. I., Metzger, D. S., Grissom, G. R., Woody, G. E., Luborsky, L., and O'Brien, C. P. (1994). Similarity of outcome predictors across opiate, cocaine, and alcohol treatments: Role of treatment services. *Journal of Consulting and Clinical Psychology* 62: 1141–58.

Mechanic, D., and Rochefort, D. A. (1990). Deinstitutionalization: An appraisal of reform. *Annual Review of Sociology* 16: 301–27

Meier, R. (1983). The impact of the structural organization of public welfare offices on the psychosocial work and treatment environments. *Journal of Social Service Research* 1: 1–18.

Milne, D. (1986). Planning and evaluating innovations in nursing practice by measuring the ward atmosphere. *Journal of Advanced Nursing* 11: 203–10.

———. (1988). Organizational behavior management in a psychiatric day hospital. *Behavioral Psychotherapy* 16: 177–78.

Moffett, L. (1984). Assessing the social system of a therapeutic community: Interpersonal orientations, social climate and norms. *International Journal of Therapeutic Communities* 5: 110–19.

Moffett, L. (1991, August). Social climates of a therapeutic community for substance dependent veterans. Paper presented at the annual meeting of the American Psychological Association, San Francisco, Calif.

Moffett, L., and Flagg, C. (1993). Real and ideal social climate perceptions of residents, staff, and visitors in a therapeutic community for substance dependent patients. *Therapeutic Communities* 14: 103–18.

Montgomery, H. A., Miller, W. R., and Tonigan, J. S. (1993). Differences among AA groups: Implications for research. *Journal of Studies on Alcohol* 54: 502–04.

Moos, R. (1968). A situational analysis of a therapeutic community milieu. *Journal of abnormal psychology* 73: 49–61.

———. (1969). Sources of variance in responses to questionnaires and in behavior. *Journal of Abnormal Psychology* 74: 405–12.

———. (1972a). Assessment of the psychosocial environments of community-oriented psychiatric treatment programs. *Journal of Abnormal Psychology* 79: 9–18.

———. (1972b). British psychiatric ward treatment environments. *British Journal of Psychiatry* 120: 635–43.

———. (1972c). Size, staffing and psychiatric ward treatment environments. *Archives of General Psychiatry* 26: 414–18.

———. (1973). Changing to the social milieus of psychiatric treatment settings. *Journal of Applied Behavioral Science* 9: 575–93.

———. (1974). *Evaluating treatment environments: A social ecological approach.* New York: Wiley.

———. (1975). *Evaluating correctional and community settings.* New York: Wiley.

———. (1979). *Evaluating educational environments: Procedures, methods, findings, and policy implications.* San Francisco: Jossey-Bass.

———. (1987). *Correctional Institutions Environment Scale manual* (2nd ed.). Palo Alto, Calif.: Mind Garden.

———. (1988). *University Residence Environment Scale manual* (2nd ed.). Palo Alto, Calif.: Mind Garden.

———. (1990). Conceptual and empirical approaches to developing family-based assessment procedures: Resolving the case of the Family Environment Scale. *Family Process* 29: 199–208.

———. (1994a). *Group Environment Scale manual* (3rd ed.). Palo Alto, Calif.: Consulting Psychologists Press.

———. (1994b). *The Social Climate Scales: A user's guide* (2nd ed.). Palo Alto, Calif.: Consulting Psychologists Press.

———. (1994c). *Work Environment Scale manual* (3rd ed.). Palo Alto, Calif.: Consulting Psychologists Press.

———. (1996a). *Community-Oriented Programs Environmental Scale manual* (3rd ed.). Palo Alto, Calif.: Mind Garden.

———. (1996b). *Ward Atmosphere Scale manual* (3rd ed.). Palo Alto, Calif.: Mind Garden.

Moos, R., and Bromet, E. (1978). Relation of patient attributes to perceptions of the treatment environment. *Journal of Consulting and Clinical Psychology* 46: 350–51.

Moos, R., and Brownstein, R. (1977). *Environment and utopia: A synthesis.* New York: Plenum.

Moos, R., and Finney, J. (in press). Effective psychosocial treatment for alcohol use disorders. In P. E. Nathan and J. M. Gorman (Eds.), *Effective treatments for DSM-IV disorders.* New York: Oxford.

Moos, R., Finney, J., and Cronkite, R. (1990). *Alcoholism treatment: Context, process, and outcome.* New York: Oxford.

Moos, R., and Houts, P. (1968). Assessment of the social atmospheres of psychiatric wards. *Journal of Abnormal Psychology* 73: 595–604.

———. (1970). Differential effects of the social atmosphere of psychiatric wards. *Human Relations* 23: 47–60.

Moos, R., King, M., and Patterson, M. (1996). Outcomes of residential treatment of substance abuse in hospital- and community-based programs. *Psychiatric Services* 47: 68–74.

Moos, R., and Lemke, S. (1994). *Group residences for older adults: Physical features, policies, and social climate.* New York: Oxford.

———. (in press). *Evaluating residential facilities.* Thousand Oaks, Calif.: Sage.

Moos, R., and MacIntosh, S. (1970). Multivariate study of the patient-therapist system: A replication and extension. *Journal of Consulting and Clinical Psychology* 35: 298–307.

Moos, R., Mehren, B., and Moos, B. (1978). Evaluation of a Salvation Army alcoholism treatment program. *Journal of Studies on Alcohol* 39: 1267–75.

Moos, R., Mertens, J., and Brennan, P. (1995). Program characteristics and readmission among older substance abuse patients: Comparisons with middle-aged and younger patients. *Journal of Mental Health Administration* 22: 332–45.

Moos, R., and Moos, B. (1994a). *Family Environment Scale manual* (3rd ed.). Palo Alto, Calif.: Consulting Psychologists Press.

———. (1994b). *Life Stressors and Social Resources Inventory Manual*. Odessa, Fla.: Psychological Assessment Resources.

Moos, R., Pettit, E., and Gruber, V. (1995a). Characteristics and outcomes of three models of community residential care for substance abuse patients. *Journal of Substance Abuse* 7: 99–116.

———. (1995b). Longer episodes of community residential care reduce substance abuse patients' readmission rates. *Journal of Studies on Alcohol* 56: 433–43.

Moos, R., and Schaefer, J. (1987). Evaluating health care work settings: A holistic conceptual framework. *Psychology and Health* 1: 97–122.

Moos, R., and Schwartz, J. (1972). Treatment environment and treatment outcome. *Journal of Nervous and Mental Diseases* 154: 264–75.

Moos, R., Shelton, R., and Petty, C. (1973). Perceived ward climate and treatment outcome. *Journal of Abnormal Psychology* 82: 291–98.

Mor, V., Sherwood, S., and Gutkin, C. (1986). A national study of residential care for the aged. *The Gerontologist* 26: 405–17.

Morgenstern, J., Frey, R. M., McCrady, B. S., Labouvie, E., and Neighbors, C. J. (1996). Examining mediators of change in traditional chemical dependency treatment. *Journal of Studies on Alcohol* 57: 53–64.

Morrissey, J. P., and Goldman, H. H. (1980). The ambiguous legacy: 1856–1968. In J. P. Morrissey, H. H. Goldman, and L. V. Klerman (Eds.), *The enduring asylum: Cycles of institutional reform at Worcester State Hospital* (45–96). New York: Grune and Stratton.

Mosher, L. R. (1991). Soteria: A therapeutic community for psychotic persons. *International Journal of Therapeutic Communities* 12: 53–67.

Mosher, L. R., and Burti, L. (1989). *Community mental health: Principles and practice*. New York: W. W. Norton and Company.

Mosher, L. R., Kesky-Wolff, M., Matthews, S., and Menn, A. (1986). Milieu therapy in the 1980s: A comparison of two residential alternatives to hospitalization. *Bulletin of the Menninger Clinic* 50: 257–68.

Mosher, L. R., and Menn, A. (1978). Lower barriers in the community: The Soteria model. In L. I. Stein and M. A. Test (Eds.), *Alternatives to mental hospital treatment* (75–113). New York: Plenum Press.

Mosher, L. R., Menn, A., and Matthews, S. (1975). Soteria: Evaluation of a home-based treatment for schizophrenia. *American Journal of Orthopsychiatry* 45: 455–67.

Murray, H. (1938). *Explorations in personality*. New York: Oxford.

Nevid, J. S., Kapurso, R., and Morrison, J. K. (1980). Patient's adjustment to family care as related to their perceptions of real-ideal differences in treatment environments. *American Journal of Community Psychology* 8: 117–20.

Ng, M. L., Tam, Y. K., and Luk, S. L. (1982). Evaluation of different forms of community meeting in a psychiatric unit in Hong Kong. *British Journal of Psychiatry* 140: 491–97.

Nissen, T. (1985). Effekten av a dele en sykehuspost for psykiatriske langtidspasienter. *Nordisk Psykiatrisk Tidsskrift* 39: 177–83.

O'Driscoll, M. P., and Evans, R. (1988). Organizational factors and perceptions of climate in three psychiatric units. *Human Relations* 41: 371–88.

O'Mahony, J. F., and Ward, M. (1995). The quality of life of chronic in-patients of a traditional psychiatric hospital in the late 1900s. *Evaluation and Program Planning* 18: 227–35.

Otto, J., and Moos, R. (1973). Evaluating descriptions of psychiatric treatment programs. *American Journal of Orthopsychiatry* 43: 401–40.

———. (1974). Patient expectations and attendance in community treatment programs. *Community Mental Health Journal* 10: 9–15.

Pallak, M. S., Cummings, N. A., Dorken, H., and Henke, C. J. (1994). Medical costs, Medicaid, and managed mental health treatment: The Hawaii study. *Managed Care Quarterly* 2: 64–70.

Patton, M. (1977). *Environments that make a difference: An evaluation of Ramsey County Corrections Foster Group Homes.* Minneapolis: University of Minnesota, Center for Social Research.

Paul, G. L. (1987). Rational operations in residential treatment settings through ongoing assessment of client and staff functioning. In D.R. Peterson and D. B. Fishman (Eds.), *Assessment For Decision* (145–203). New Brunswick, N.J.: Rutgers University Press.

Paul, G. L., and Lentz, R. J. (1977). *Psychosocial treatment of chronic mental patients: Milieu versus social-learning programs.* Cambridge, Mass.: Harvard University Press.

Paul, G. L., and Menditto, A. A. (1992). Effectiveness of inpatient treatment programs for mentally ill adults in public psychiatric facilities. *Applied and Preventive Psychology* 1: 41–63.

Pendorf, J. E. (1990). Vocational rehabilitation for psychiatric in-patient Vietnam combat veterans. *Military Medicine* 155: 369–71.

Penk, W., and Robinowitz, R. (1978). Drug users' views of psychosocial aspects of their treatment environment. *Drug Forum* 7: 129–43.

Peterson, K. A., Swindle, R. W., Phibbs, C. S., Recine, B., and Moos, R. H. (1994). Determinants of readmission following inpatient substance abuse treatment: A national study of VA programs. Medical Care 32: 535–50.

Pierce, W., Trickett, E., and Moos, R. (1972). Changing ward atmosphere through staff discussion of the perceived ward environment. *Archives of General Psychiatry* 26: 35–41.

Pinel, P. (1806). *A treatise on insanity* (D. D. Davis, trans.). London. Todd, Sheffield.

Pino, C. J., and Howard, S. (1984). Sex differences in environmental perceptions, activities and behavior mapping in well-aged housing residents. *Journal of Gerontological Social Work* 6: 3–17.

Po, K. M. (1989). An investigation of the program performance of black women in a multimodal drug rehabilitation facility (Doctoral dissertation, Columbia University, 1988). *Dissertations Abstracts International* 50: 1118.

Polich, J. M., Armor, D. J., and Braiker, H. B. (1981). *The course of alcoholism: Four years after treatment.* New York: Wiley.

Pratt, R., Linn, M., Carmichael, J., and Webb, N. (1977). The alcoholic's perception of the ward as a predictor of aftercare attendance. *Journal of Clinical Psychology* 33: 915–18.

Price, R., and Moos, R. (1975). Toward a taxonomy of inpatient treatment environments. *Journal of Abnormal Psychology* 84: 181–88.

Pullen, G. P. (1982). Street: The 17 day community. *International Journal of Therapeutic Communities* 2: 115–26.

———. (1986). The Eric Burden Community. *International Journal of Therapeutic Communities* 7: 191–200.

Pullen, G., and Clark, D. (1983). What tune are we marching to? Teamwork in a rehabilitation service. *International Journal of Therapeutic Communities* 2: 115–26.

Rapaport, R. (1960). *Community as doctor.* London: Tavistock.

Raush, H., and Raush, C. (1968). *The halfway house movement: A search for sanity.* New York: Appleton-Century-Crofts.

Redick, R. W., Witkin, M. J., Atay, J. E., and Manderscheid, R. W. (1994). Highlights of organized mental health services in 1990 and major national and state trends. In R. W. Manderscheid and M. A. Sonnensehein (Eds.), *Mental Health, United States* (77–125) (DHHS Pub. No. SMA 94-3000). Washington, D.C.: U. S. Government Printing Office.

Rhodes, L. (1981). Social climate perception and depression of patients and staff in a chronic hemodialysis unit. *Journal of Nervous and Mental Disease* 169: 169–75.

Rosenfield, S. (1992). Factors contributing to the subjective quality of life of the chronic mentally ill. *Journal of Health and Social Behavior* 33: 299–315.

Rosenheck, R., Frisman, L., and Gallup, P. (1995). Effectiveness and cost of specific treatment elements in a program for homeless mentally ill veterans. *Psychiatric Services* 46: 1131–39.

Rutman, I. D. (1987). The psychosocial rehabilitation movement in the United States. In A. Meyerson and T. Find (Eds.), *Psychiatric Disability* (197–220). Washington, D.C.: American Psychiatric Association Press.

Ryan, E., and Bell, M. (1983). Follow-up of a psychoanalytically oriented long-term treatment program for schizophrenic inpatients. *American Journal of Orthopsychiatry* 53: 730–39.

Ryan, E., Bell, M., and Metcalf, J. (1982). The development of a rehabilitation psychology program for schizophrenics: Changes in the treatment environment. *Rehabilitation Psychology* 27: 67–85.

Sanders, R., Smith, R., and Weinman, B. (1967). *Chronic psychoses and recovery: An experiment in socio-environmental treatment.* San Francisco: Jossey-Bass.

Schaefer, J. A., and Moos, R. H. (1993). Relationship, task, and system stressors in the health care workplace. *Journal of Community and Applied Social Psychology* 3: 285–98.

———. (1996). Effects of work stressors and work climate on long-term care staff's job morale and functioning. *Research in Nursing and Health* 19: 63–73.

Schlesinger, M., and Dorwart, R. (1984). Ownership and mental health services: A reappraisal of the shift toward privately owned facilities. *New England Journal of Medicine* 311: 959–65.

Schmidt, J., Wakefield, D., and Andersen, C. (1979). Ward atmosphere: A longitudinal and factorial analysis. *Social Psychiatry* 14: 119–23.

Schmidt, J. P., Thorarenson, D., Buchberger, G., Abernethy, J., and Zakos, B. (1980). Issues in psychiatric day care programs in nonurban areas: A case study. *Canada's Mental Health* 28: 13–14, 20.

Schmidt, L., and Weisner, C. (1993). Developments in Alcoholism. In M. Galanter, (Ed.), *Recent developments in alcoholism: Ten years of progress* (Vol. 2, 364–96). New York: Plenum.

Schneider, K., Kinlow, M. R., Galloway, A. N., and Ferro, D. L. (1982). An analysis of the effects of implementing the teaching/family model in two community based group homes. *Child Care Quarterly* 11: 298–311.

Sechrest, L., West, S., Phillips, M., Redner, R., and Yeaton, W. (1979). Some neglected problems in evaluation research: Strength and integrity of treatments. In L. Sechrest, S. West, M. Phillips, R. Redner, and W. Yeaton (Eds.), *Evaluation studies review annual* (Vol. 4, 15–35). Beverly Hills, Calif.: Sage.

Segal, S., and Aviram, U. (1978). *The mentally ill in community-based sheltered care: A study of community care and social integration.* New York: Wiley.

Segal, S., Everett-Dille, L., and Moyles, E. (1979). Congruent perceptions in the evaluation of community care facilities. *Journal of Community Psychology* 7: 60–68.

Segal, S., and Holschuh, J. (1991). Effects of sheltered care environments and resident characteristics on the development of social networks. *Hospital and Community Psychiatry* 42: 1125–31.

Segal, S. P., and Kotler, P. (1989). Community residential care. In D. A. Rochefort, (Ed.), *Handbook on mental health policy in the United States* (237–65). Westport, Conn.: Greenwood.

Segal, S., and Moyles, E. (1979). Management style and institutional dependency in sheltered care. *Social Psychiatry* 14: 159–65.

Seligman, M. E. (1995). The effectiveness of psychotherapy: The consumer reports study. *American Psychologist* 50: 965–74.

Shadish, W. R. (1989). Private-sector care for chronically mentally ill individuals: The more things change, the more they stay the same. *American Psychologist* 44: 1142–47.

Shadish, W. R., Orwin, R. G., Silber, B. G., and Bootzin, R.R. (1985). The subjective well-being of mental patients in nursing homes. *Evaluation and Program Planning* 8: 239–50.

Shealy, C. N. (1995). From Boys Town to Oliver Twist: Separating fact from fiction in welfare reform and out-of-home placement of children and youth. *American Psychologist* 50: 565–80.

Shinn, M. (1982). Assessing program characteristics and social climate. In A. J. McSweeny, R. Hawkins, and W. Fremouw (Eds.), *Practical program evaluation in youth treatment* (116–43). Springfield, Ill.: Charles Thomas.

Shinn, M., Perkins, D., and Cherniss, C. (1980). Using survey-guided development to improve program climates: An experimental evaluation in group homes for youths. In R. Stough and A. Wandersman (Eds.), *Optimizing environments: Research, practice and policy* (124–35). New York: Environmental Design Research Association.

Sidman, J., and Moos, R. (1973). On the relation between psychiatric ward atmosphere and helping behavior. *Journal of Clinical Psychology* 29: 74–78.

Sinclair, C., and Frankel, M. (1982). The effect of quality assurance activities on the quality of mental health services. *Quality Review Bulletin* 8: 7–15.

Slater, E., and Linn, M. (1982-83). Predictors of rehospitalization in a male alcoholic population. *American Journal of Drug and Alcohol Abuse* 9: 211–20.

Smith, W. R., and Grant, B. L. (1989). Effects of a smoking ban on a general hospital psychiatric service. *Hospital and Community Psychiatry* 40: 497–502.

Solzhenitsyn, A. (1969). *Cancer ward.* New York: Bantam Books.

Sommers, I. (1987). Tolerance of deviance and the community adjustment of the mentally ill. *Community Mental Health Journal* 23: 159–72.

Sparr, L. F., Ruud, D. H., Hickam, D. H., and Cooney, T. G. (1994). The effect of house officer rotation on inpatient satisfaction and ward atmosphere: Preliminary findings. *Military Medicine* 159: 47–53.

Spencer, J. H., Jr., Glick, I. D., Haas, G. L., Clarkin, J. F., Lewis, A. B., Peyser, J., DeMane, N., Good-Ellis, M., Harris, E., and Lestelle, V. (1988). A randomized clinical trial of inpatient family intervention. III: Effects at 6-month and 18-month follow-ups. *American Journal of Psychiatry* 145: 1115–21.

Squier, R. W. (1994). The relationship between ward atmosphere and staff attitude to treatment in psychiatric in-patient units. *British Journal of Medical Psychology* 67: 319–31.

Stanton, A., Gunderson, J. G., Knapp, P. H., Frank, A. F., Vannicelli, M. L., Schnitzer, R., and Rosenthal, R. (1984). Effects of psychotherapy in schizophrenia: I. Design and implementation of a controlled study. *Schizophrenia Bulletin* 10: 520–63.

Stanton, A., and Schwartz, M. (1954). *The mental hospital: A study of institutional participation in psychiatric illness and treatment.* New York: Basic Books.

Starker, S. (1989). Working up to a better workplace. *VA Practitioner* 6: 33–44.

Stein, L. (1989). The community as the primary locus of care for persons with serious long-term mental illness. In G. M. Bonjean, M. T. Coleman, and I. Iscoe (Eds.), *Community care of the mentally ill* (11–29). Austin, Tex.: Hogg Foundation for Mental Health.

Steiner, H. (1982). The sociotherapeutic environment of a child psychosomatic ward (or, Is pediatrics bad for your mental health?). *Child Psychiatry and Human Development* 13: 71–78.

Steiner, H., Haldipur, C., and Stack, L. (1982). The acute admission ward as a therapeutic community. *American Journal of Psychiatry* 139: 897–901.

Steiner, H., Marx, L., and Walton, C. (1991). The ward atmosphere of a child psychosomatic unit: A ten year follow-up. *General Hospital Psychiatry* 13: 1–7.

Stern, G. (1970). *People in context: Measuring person-environment congruence in education and industry.* New York: Wiley.

Stirling, G., and Reid, D. W. (1992). The application of participatory control to facilitate patient well-being: An experimental study of nursing impact on geriatric patients. *Canadian Journal of Behavioral Science* 24: 204–19.

Stotland, E., and Kobler, A. (1965). *Life and death of a mental hospital.* Seattle: University of Washington Press.

Strasser, D. C., Falconer, J. A., Martino-Saltzman, D. (1992). The relationship of patient's age to the perceptions of the rehabilitation environment. *Journal of the American Geriatrics Society* 40: 445–48.

———. (1994). The rehabilitation team: Staff perceptions of the hospital environment, the interdisciplinary team environment, and interprofessional relations. *Archives of Physical Medicine Rehabilitation* 75: 177–82.

Sugarman, B. (1974). *Daytop Village: A therapeutic community.* New York: Holt, Rinehart, and Winston.

Swindle, R., Peterson, K., Paradise, M., and Moos, R. (1995). Measuring program treatment orientations: The drug and alcohol treatment inventory. *Journal of Substance Abuse* 7: 79–97.

Swindle, R., Phibbs, C., Paradise, M., Recine, B., and Moos, R. (1995). Inpatient treatment for substance abuse patients with psychiatric disorders: A national study of determinants of readmission. *Journal of Substance Abuse* 7: 79–97.

Talbott, J. A. (1988). Nursing homes are not the answer. *Hospital and Community Psychiatry* 39: 115.

Terry, K., Sobieski, J., Dunne, K., and Steiner, H. (1984). A comparison of staff and patient perceptions of a child and adolescent psychosomatic unit and a pediatric unit. *Child Psychiatry and Human Development* 14: 230–48.

Tessier, W. G. (1990). The impact of ward atmosphere on patient discharge status from locked psychiatric units (Doctoral dissertation, Boston College, 1988). *Dissertation Abstracts International* 50: 3178.

Thomas, L. H. (1992). Qualified nurse and nursing auxiliary perceptions of their work environment in primary, team, and functional nursing wards. *Journal of Advanced Nursing* 17: 373–82.

Thorward, S. R., and Birnbaum, S. (1989). Effects of a smoking ban on a general hospital psychiatric unit. *General Hospital Psychiatry* 11: 63–67.

Timko, C. (1995). Policies and services in residential substance abuse programs: Comparisons with psychiatric programs. *Journal of Substance Abuse* 7: 43–59.

———. (1996). Physical characteristics of residential psychiatric and substance abuse programs: Organizational determinants and patients' outcomes. *American Journal of Community Psychology* 24.

Timko, C., Finney, J., and Moos, B. (1995). Short-term treatment careers and outcomes of previously untreated alcoholics. *Journal of Studies on Alcohol* 56: 597–610.

Timko, C., and Moos, R. (1990). Determinants of support and self-direction in group residential facilities for the elderly. *Journals of Gerontology* 45: S184–S192.

———. (1996). *Determinants of social climate in residential psychiatric and substance abuse treatment programs.* Palo Alto, Calif.: Department of Veteran Affairs, Center for Health Care Evaluation.

Timko, C., Nguyen, A. T., Williford, W. O., and Moos, R. (1993). Quality of care and chronically mentally ill patients' outcomes in hospitals and nursing homes. *Hospital and Community Psychiatry* 44: 241–46.

Tommasini, N. R. (1992). The impact of a staff support group on the work environment of a specialty unit. *Archives of Psychiatric Nursing* 6: 40–47.

Trauer, T., Bouras, N., and Watson, J. P. (1987). The assessment of ward atmosphere in a psychiatric unit. *International Journal of Therapeutic Communities* 8: 199–205.

Vaglum, P., Friis, S., Irion, T., Johns, S., Karterud, S., Larsen, F., and Vaglum, S. (1990). Treatment response of severe and nonsevere personality disorders in a therapeutic community day unit. *Journal of Personality Disorders* 4: 161–72.

Vaglum, P., Friis, S., and Karterud, S. (1985). Why are the results of milieu therapy for schizophrenic patients contradictory? An analysis based on four empirical studies. *The Yale Journal of Biology and Medicine* 58: 349–61.

Van Stone, W., and Gilbert, R. (1972). Peer confrontation groups–what, why and whether. *American Journal of Psychiatry* 129: 583–89.

Verhaest, S. (1983). The assessment of the maturation of a therapeutic community. *International Journal of Therapeutic Communities* 4: 183–95.

Verhaest, S., Pierloot, R., and Janssens, G. (1982). Comparative assessment of two different types of therapeutic communities. *International Journal of Social Psychiatry* 28: 46–52.

Verinis, J. (1983). Ward atmosphere as a factor in irregular discharge for an alcohol rehabilitation unit. *International Journal of the Addictions* 18: 895–99.

Verinis, J., and Flaherty, J. (1978). Using the Ward Atmosphere Scale to help change the treatment environment. *Hospital and Community Psychiatry* 29: 238–40.

Walz, L. T., and Goldstein, L. H. (1992). The mental impairment and evaluation treatment service: Staff attitudes and staff-client interactions. *Psychological Medicine* 22: 503–11.

Ward, M. J. (1946). *The snake pit.* New York: Random House.

Waxman, H., Carner, E., and Berkenstock, G. (1984). Job turnover and job satisfaction among nursing home aides. *The Gerontologist* 24: 503–09.

Wechsler, H. (1960). Halfway houses for former mental patients: A survey. *Journal of Social Issues* 16: 20–26.

Weinstein, R. (1979). Patient attitudes toward mental hospitalization: A review of quantitative research. *Journal of Health and Social Behavior* 20: 237–58.

Wendt, R., Mosher, L., Matthews, S., and Menn, A. (1983). Comparison of two treatment environments for schizophrenia. In J. G. Gunderson, O. A. Will, and L. R. Mosher (Eds.), *Principles and practice of milieu therapy* (17–33). New York: Aronson.

Wilder, J., Kessell, M., and Caulfield, S. (1968). Follow-up of a high expectations halfway house. *American Journal of Psychiatry* 124: 103–09.

Wilderman, R., and Mezzelo, J. (1984). Paving the road to financial security: The direct service model. *Administration in Mental Health* 11: 184–94.

Willer, B. (1977). Individualized patient programming: An experiment in the use of evaluation and feedback for hospital psychiatry. *Evaluation Quarterly* 1: 587–608.

Willer, B., and Intagliata, J. (1981). Social environmental factors as predictors of adjustment of deinstitutionalized mentally retarded adults. *American Journal of Mental Deficiency* 86: 252–59.

———. (1984). *Promises and realities for mentally retarded citizens: Life in the community.* Baltimore, Md.: University Park Press.

Wilson, W. T. (1993). The influence of staff and organizational characteristics on social environment in substance abuse treatment facilities (Doctoral dissertation, The University of Texas Health Science Center at Houston School of Public Health, 1992). *Dissertations Abstracts International* 54: 769.

Wing, J., and Brown, G. (1970). *Institutionalism and schizophrenia: A comparative study of three mental hospitals, 1960–1968.* London: Cambridge University Press.

Winnett, R. L. (1989). Long-term care reconsidered: The role of the psychologist in the geriatric rehabilitation milieu. *Journal of Applied Gerontology* 8, 53-68.

Wolf, M. (1978). The effect of education on nurses' views of a therapeutic milieu. *Journal of Psychiatric Nursing* 16: 29–33.

Wolff, W., Herrin, B., Scarborough, D., Wiggins, K., and Winman, F. (1972). Integration of an instructional program with a psychotherapeutic milieu: Developmental redirection for seriously disturbed children. *Acta Paedopsychiatrica* 39: 83–92.

Woods, D., and Billig, J. (1979). The A-B variable and preferred inpatient environment. *Journal of Clinical Psychology* 35: 429–32.

Yates, B. T. (1995). Cost-effectiveness analysis, cost-benefit analysis, and beyond: Evolving models of scientist-manager-practitioner. *Clinical Psychology: Science and Practice* 2: 385–98.

Yeaton, W. H., and Sechrest, L. (1981). Critical dimensions in the choice and maintenance of successful treatments: Strength, integrity, and effectiveness. *Journal of Consulting and Clinical Psychology* 49: 156–67.

Zillmer, E. W., Archer, R. P., and Glidden, R. A. (1986). Ward atmosphere perception: Relationship to job training and experience, demographic features, and locus of control. *Journal of Social and Clinical Psychology* 4: 142–53.

Author Index

Abernethy, J.: 54
Abramowitz, S.: 161
Acrish, W.P.: 163
Alden, L.: 36, 185
Alexy, W.: 76
Allen, C.: 93, 153
Allen, J.P.: 225
Allen, K.: 226
Alper, B.: 92
Alterman, A.I.: 70
Amaral, P.: 231
Andersen, C.: 37, 53, 54
Appelbaum, A.H.: 124
Apte, R.: 92, 93
Archer, R.P.: 41
Armor, D.J.: 200
Arrington, B.: 159
Atay, J.E.: 11
Austin, J.K.: 41
Aviram, U.: 209, 210, 225
Azrin, N.: 250

Baird, J.W.: 41, 76
Bakos, M.: 174
Baldwin, S.: 163
Bale, R.: 192, 207
Ballinari, P.: 72
Barchiesi, A.: 221
Barker, R.T.: 66
Barker, S.B.: 66
Barlow, J.: 42
Bass, A.: 193
Bausell, R.B.: 153
Beard, J.H.: 93
Belknap, I.: 10
Bell, M.: 122, 123, 124, 137, 142, 190
Berglund, M.: 42, 188
Berkenstock, G.: 228
Berman, A.: 215

Bernstein, E.: 72
Billig, J.: 43
Birnbaum, S.: 53
Bjorkman, T.: 42
Blacker, E.: 91
Blackwell, C.C.: 56
Bliss, F.: 117
Blotcky, M.J.: 200
Bocker, F.M.: 181
Bootzin, R.R.: 220, 221
Bouras, N.: 75
Bowman, R.G.: 53
Boyd, M.A.: 66
Boydell, K.M.: 142
Bozic, R.: 174
Bradshaw, S.: 55
Braiker, H.B.: 200
Brennan, P.: 205, 229
Bromet, E.: 103, 117
Brown, G.: 8, 9
Brown, P.: 10
Brownstein, R.: 16
Buchberger, G.: 54
Burda, P.C.: 72
Burti, L.: 152
Bushey, M.: 58

Cahn, S.: 92
Caplan, C.A.: 75
Carmichael, J.: 193
Carner, E.: 228
Carroll, R.S.: 67
Casey, D.: 163
Casey, N.: 218, 219
Caudill, W.: 7, 8
Caulfield, S.: 92
Chabloz, D.: 212
Chapin, D.: 174
Chappuis, J.: 212

Cherniss, C.: 129
Christenfeld, R.: 163
Clark, D.: 72
Clark, R.E.: 247
Clarkin, J.F.: 206
Cochran, M.: 36
Cohen, P.: 188
Cohen, R.: 92
Cohen, S.: 219
Colligan, R.C.: 77
Collins, J.: 218, 219
Comstock, B.S.: 141
Connors, G.J.: 225
Cook, C.: 208
Cooney, T.G.: 53
Cooper, L.: 64
Corey, L.J.: 163
Costello, R.: 36
Coulton, C.J.: 224
Coyne, L.: 188, 200
Cressler, D.: 13, 93
Crisler, J.: 77
Cronkite, R.: 4, 70, 103, 117, 115, 136,
    199, 213, 220, 249
Cruser, D.A.: 70, 71
Culhane, D.P.: 159
Cummings, N.A.: 244
Curtiss, S.: 54

Dassen, T.: 185
Dauwalder, J.: 212
Davis, R.C.: 181
Dayson, D.: 149
Deering, C.D.: 188, 200
DeLeon, G.: 92
DeMane, N.: 206
Denny, N.: 36
De-Nour, A.K.: 76
Desiderato, O.: 41
Devlin, A.S.: 162
Dickens, C.: 5
Dickie, E.: 187
Dimperio, T.L.: 200
Doherty, E.: 194
Dominguez, F. 72
Doniger, J.: 92
Dorken, H.: 244
Dorr, D.: 228
Dorwart, R.: 159
Downs, M.W.: 148
Drake, R.E.: 247

Dunne, K.: 78

Eckert, A.: 66
Edlund, M.J.: 247
Egerter, E.: 187
Ejsing, L.O.: 65
Elashoff, R.: 192, 207
Elliott, B.: 187
Ellsworth, R.: 23, 195, 196, 200, 218,
    219
Elpers, R.: 92, 114
Elzinga, R.H.: 42
Engelsing, T.: 192, 207
Eriksen, L.: 53
Erikson, E.: 7
Erlangen: 57
Evans, R.: 28, 227
Everett, B.: 142
Everett-Dille, L.: 209

Fairchild, H.: 181, 228
Fairweather, G.: 12, 13, 93, 250
Fakhouri, J.: 151
Falconer, J.A.: 39, 76, 77
Farndale, J.: 92
Feist, J.R.: 77
Fernandez, E.: 72
Ferro, D.L.: 122
Finnema, E.J.: 185
Finney, J.: 4, 70, 117, 131, 136, 152,
    199, 213, 244, 249, 250, 251
Firth, H.: 66
Fischer, J.: 36, 212
Fitch, V.: 224
Flagg, C.: 73
Flaherty, J.: 39, 59
Flannery, R.B.: 185
Fontana, A.: 162, 192
Fox, J.C.: 148
Fox, L.: 231
Frank, A.F.: 72
Frank, R.G.: 247
Frankel, M.: 230
Frey, R.M.: 251
Friedman, A.S.: 104, 153, 191, 208
Friedman, S: 41, 59, 130
Friis, S.: 28, 36, 41, 65, 66, 75, 161, 162,
    168, 171, 172, 186, 193, 196, 216,
    217, 223, 228
Frisman, L.: 248, 249

Galloway, A.N.: 122
Gallup, P.: 248, 249
Garety, P.A.: 93, 153
Geller, J.L.: 149
Gift, T.E.: 74
Gilbert, R.: 73
Gillespie, C.R.: 93, 153
Glasscote, R.: 92, 114
Glassman, S.: 114
Glick, I.D.: 72, 152, 206
Glickman, N.W.: 104, 153, 191, 208
Glidden, R.A.: 41
Godley, M.: 250
Goertzel, V.: 92
Goffman, E.: 8, 10
Goldberg, A.: 215
Goldman, H.H.: 10
Goldmeier, J.: 171
Goldstein, J.M: 188
Goldstein, L.H.: 149, 153
Gooch, C.: 149
Good-Ellis, M.: 206
Gordon, H.: 23, 159, 196, 200
Gossett, J.T.: 200
Gotestam, K.G.: 55
Grame, C.J.: 188, 200
Grant, B.L.: 53
Grant, R.: 48
Greenberg, E.: 40
Greenberg, J.: 9
Greene, L.: 161
Gripp, R.: 53
Grissom, G.R.: 70
Grob, G.: 6
Growe, G.: 219
Gruber, V.: 70, 245, 248
Gudeman, J.: 92, 114
Gunderson, J.G.: 72, 178
Gunn, R.: 23, 195, 196, 200
Gurel, L.: 221
Gurland, B.: 221
Gutkin, C.: 11

Haas, G.L.: 206
Haddock, C.C.: 159
Hadley, T.R.: 159
Hahn, A.: 152
Haldipur, C.: 75, 78
Halfens, R.: 185
Halford, W.K.: 243, 249
Hall, J.N.: 93, 153

Hall, S.: 193
Hanson, M.A.: 185
Hansson, L.: 42, 188
Harder, D.W.: 74
Hargreaves, W.: 72, 193
Harris, E.: 206
Harris, R.: 193
Harris, S.H.: 163
Hartmann, H.: 7
Hattie, J.A.: 136
Hayes, R.: 243, 249
Heim, E.: 72
Hellman, I.: 161
Henke, C.J.: 244
Herrera, J.M.: 65
Herrin, B.: 77
Hickam, D.H.: 53
Hickey, R.: 218, 219
Hicks, C.: 185
Hills, A.A.: 59
Hippius, H.: 57
Hoare, C.: 42, 179
Holland, J.: 168
Holland, T.E.: 224
Holschuh, J.: 210
Honea, S.: 228
Houts, P.: 35, 39, 181, 182
Howard, S.: 103
Humphreys, K.: 228
Hyer, L.: 218, 219

Ingstad, J.: 55
Intagliata, J.: 169, 211, 212
Irion, T.: 41, 193

Jackson, J.: 23
James, I.: 66
Jansen, E.: 100, 101
Janssens, G.: 74
Jeger, A.: 41, 59, 130
Jepson, W.: 114
Johns, S.: 41, 193
Johnson, S.: 227
Jones, M.: 11, 25, 207

Kadden, R.M.: 225
Kahn, E.M.: 186, 219
Kamiliar, S.M.: 141
Kanter, R.M.: 91
Kantor, D.: 91
Kaplan, H.B.: 141

Kapurso, R.: 224
Karterud, S.: 41, 66, 193, 217
Kaufbeuren: 57
Kaye, D.: 40
Kayne, H.L.: 185
Kellam, S.: 215
Keller, O.: 92
Kelly, G.R.: 59
Kennard, D.: 6, 207
Kesey, K.: 9, 25
Kesky-Wolff, M.: 151
Keso, L.: 190, 208
Kessell, M.: 92
Kessler, R.C.: 247
Khan, A.: 219
King, M.: 142
King, R.: 23
Kinlow, M.R.: 122
Kish, G.: 40, 41, 59, 71
Klass, D.: 219
Klein, R.: 58
Kleppe, H.: 66
Klett, W.: 23, 159, 196, 200
Knapp, P.H.: 72
Kobler, A.: 8
Kobos, J.: 37
Koenig, G.: 36
Kokes, R.F.: 74
Koran, L.: 231
Kotler, P.: 11
Kovach, J.A.: 104, 153, 208
Kraft, A.: 114
Kuldau, J.: 192, 207
Kyrouz, E.: 228

Labouvie, E.: 251
Lacoursiere, R.: 55
Lamb, R.: 91, 92
Landy, D.: 92
Langenbucher, J.: 244
Langworthy, D.E.: 188, 200
Lanza, M.L.: 185
Larsen, F.: 41, 193
Laughlin, P.: 221
Lavender, A.: 66
Lawson, W.B.: 65
Lawton, M.P.: 216, 222
Lawton, R.: 39, 59
Leaf, P.J.: 247
Leda, C.: 141, 162, 192
Leff, J.: 149

Lehman, A.F.: 74, 179, 218, 220
Leiberich, P.: 55
Lemke, S.: 40, 159, 161, 163, 164, 165, 170, 186, 223
Lentz, R.J.: 15
Lestelle, V.: 206
Leutje, V.: 66
Leviege, V.: 57
Lewis, A.B.: 206
Lewis, S.A.: 188
Liberman, R.P.: 92
Lieberman, P.B.: 187
Lindsay, J.S.B.: 75
Linn, M.: 11, 39, 137, 194, 212, 221
Linton, R.: 17
Lipsey, M.: 244
Loeb, P.: 193
Long, C.G.: 56
Longabaugh, R.: 225
Lorentzen, S.: 66
Luborsky, L.: 70
Luft, L.: 151
Luk, S.L.: 53
Lystrup, S.: 66

MacDonald, L.: 42, 179
MacInnes, M.: 53
MacIntosh, S.: 17
Magaro, P.: 53
Main, S.: 41
Makkai, T.: 38
Malamud, T.J.: 93
Mandersheid, R.W.: 11, 36
Mann, T.: 9
Manning, N.: 141
Marone, J.: 41
Maroney, R.: 23, 195, 196, 200
Martino-Saltzman, D.: 39, 76, 77
Marx, L.: 78
Matthews, S.: 150, 151
Mattson, M.E.: 225
Maynard, H.: 13, 93
McAllister, I.: 38
McBride, A.B.: 41
McCrady, B.S.: 251
McFarlane, W.J.G.: 53
McGee, M.: 77
McGlashan, T.H.: 200
McGonagle, K.A.: 247
McKenna, H.: 57
McLellan, A.T.: 70

McSweeny, A.J.: 220
Mechanic, D.: 10
Medak, S.: 141
Mehren, B.: 193
Meier, R.: 227
Menditto, A.A.: 178, 243
Menn, A.: 150, 151
Mertens, J.: 205
Metcalf, J.: 123
Metzger, D.S.: 70
Meyers, R.: 250
Mezzelo, J.: 230
Midgley, M.: 56
Miller, A.: 67
Miller, W.R.: 136
Milne, D.L.: 65, 66
Milner, J.: 185
Moffett, L.: 72, 73, 139
Monahan, S.: 244
Montgomery, H.A.: 136
Moos, B.: 105, 193, 211, 231, 244, 250
Mor, V.: 11
Morgenstern, J.: 251
Morris, I.: 93, 153
Morrison, J.K.: 224
Morrison, T.: 161
Morrissey, J.P.: 10
Mosher, L.R.: 150, 151, 152
Moyles, E.: 161, 209, 210
Mueser, K.T.: 247
Munchen: 57
Munich, R.L.: 124
Murray, H.: 24, 25
Myers, C.P.: 179

Naidu, J.: 39, 59
Nehemkis, A.: 231
Neighbors, C.J.: 251
Nelson, C.B.: 247
Nesselroade, J.: 218
Neuman, S.: 174
Nevid, J.S.: 224
Ng, M.L.: 53
Nguyen, A.T.: 221, 222
Nickless, C.J.: 225
Nissen, T.: 161

Obitz, F.: 40
O'Brien, C.P.: 70
O'Driscoll, M.P.: 28, 227
Olson, R.: 141

O'Mahoney, J.F.: 179
Orwin, R.G.: 221
Otto, J.: 113, 187
Overall, J.: 221

Pallak, M.S.: 244
Paradise, M.J.: 141, 188, 193, 205, 206, 245, 247
Pastva, G: 163
Pathak, D.: 39
Patterson, M.: 142
Patton, M.: 192
Paul, G.L.: 15, 178, 243, 251
Pendorf, J.E.: 72
Penk, W.E.: 139, 185
Perkins, D.: 129
Peterson, K.A.: 188, 193, 206
Pettit, E.: 70, 245, 248
Petty, C.: 189
Peyser, J.: 206
Phibbs, C.S.: 188, 193, 206
Phillips, M.: 70, 131
Pierce, W.: 61
Pierloot, R.: 74
Pilsbury, J.: 58
Pinel, P.: 5
Pino, C.J.: 103
Po, K.M.: 220
Polich, J.M.: 200
Pozner, R.: 228
Pratt, R.: 193
Pratt, T.: 193, 194
Price, R.: 75, 78
Propst, R.N.: 93
Pullen, G.P.: 72, 75

Ramirez, J.V.: 141
Rapaport, R.: 12, 249
Raush, H.: 92
Raush, C.: 92
Raynes, N.: 23
Recine, B.: 188, 193, 206
Redick, R.W.: 11
Redmond, F.: 37
Redner, R.: 70, 131
Reid, D.W.: 57, 227
Rhodes, L.: 76
Rinkus, A.: 153
Ritzler, B.A.: 74, 218, 220
Robinowitz, R.: 139
Rochefort, D.A.: 10

Rogers, H.J.: 136
Rooks, T.E.: 188, 200
Rosenfield, S.: 211, 221
Rosenheck, R.: 141, 162, 192, 248, 249
Rosenthal, R.: 72
Ross, B.: 67
Rothwell, N.: 92
Rutman, I.D.: 92
Ruud, D.H.: 53
Ryan, E.: 122, 123, 124

Salaspuro, M.: 190, 208
Sanders, D.: 13, 93
Sanders, R.: 14
Saslow, G.: 48
Scarborough, D.: 77
Schaefer, J.: 4, 227
Schaeffer, J.: 186
Schlesinger, M.: 159
Schmelzer, J.: 215
Schmidt, J.P.: 37, 53, 54
Schmidt, L.: 247
Schneider, K.: 122
Schnitzer, R.: 72
Schooler, N.: 215
Schoonover, R.: 218
Schwartz, J.: 189, 203
Schwartz, M.: 7
Sechrest, L.: 70, 71, 131
Segal, S.: 11, 161, 209, 210, 225
Seligman, M.E.: 244
Settles, R.: 77
Shadish, W.R.: 159, 220, 221
Shane, R: 194
Sharpley, C.F.: 136
Shealy, C.N.: 122
Shelton, R.: 189
Sheppard, G.: 215
Sherwood, S.: 11
Shinn, M.: 129, 130
Sibbald, B.: 42, 179
Sidman, J.: 183
Silber, B.G.: 221
Silbergeld, S.: 36
Silver, S.B.: 171
Simpson, G.M.: 67
Sinclair, C.: 230
Sisson, R.: 250
Slater, E.: 212
Slaughter, J.G.: 179
Slotnick, R.: 41, 59, 130

Slowiak, C.A.: 77
Smith, W.R.: 53
Smith, M.J.: 188, 200
Smith, R.: 14
Snell, S.: 58
Sobieski, J.: 78
Solberg, K.: 40, 41
Solzhenitsyn, A.: 9
Sommers, I.: 206
Sparr, L.F.: 53
Spencer, J.H., Jr.: 206
Spohn, H.E.: 188, 200
Squier, R.W.: 36, 41, 75, 196
Stack, L.: 75, 78
Stanton, A.: 7, 72
Starker, S.: 227
Starkey: T.W.: 72
Stein, L.: 91
Stein, S.: 11
Steiner, H.: 75, 77, 78
Sterling, J.: 37
Stern, G.: 24, 25
Stirling, G.: 57, 227
Storke, I.T.: 186
Stotland, E.: 8
Strasser, D.C.: 39, 76, 77
Strauss, J.S.: 74
Strizich, M.: 219
Struening, E.L.: 188
Sugarman, B.: 92
Swindle, R.W.: 141, 188, 193, 205, 206,
   245, 247

Talbott, J.A.: 221
Tam, Y.K.: 53
Tansella, M.: 152
Taylor, M.W.: 188, 200
Terry, K.: 78
Tessier, W.G.: 193
Thomas, L.H.: 231
Thorarenson, D.: 54
Thornby, J.I.: 141
Thornicroft, G.: 149
Thorward, S.R.: 53
Timko, C.: 100, 140, 149, 157, 158, 159,
   161, 162, 165, 166, 167, 170, 171,
   172, 173, 221, 222, 244, 246
Tommasini, N.R.: 231
Tonigan, J.S.: 136
Trauer, T.: 75
Trickett, E.: 61

Twemlow, S.: 218

Uecker, A.: 40, 41

Vaglum, P.: 41, 193, 217
Vaglum, S.: 41, 66, 193
Vannicelli, M.L.: 72
Van Stone, W.: 73, 192, 207
Verhaest, S.: 53, 55, 74
Verinis, J.: 59, 64, 188
Verinis, S.: 59
Von Rehn, S.: 187
Von Cranach, M.: 57

Wagner, J.: 163
Wakefield, D.: 37, 53, 54
Wallace, M.A.: 163
Wallach, M.A.: 247
Walton, C.: 78
Walz, L.T.: 149, 153
Ward, M.: 179
Ward, M.J.: 9, 25
Watson, D.: 153
Watson, J.P.: 75
Waxman, H.: 228
Webb, N.: 193, 194
Wechsler, H.: 92
Weinman, B.: 14
Weinstein, R.: 179

Weisner, C.: 247
Wendt, R.: 150
West, S.: 70, 131
White, E.M.: 219
Wiggins, K.: 77
Wilder, J.: 92
Wilderman, R.: 230
Willer, B.: 53, 54, 169, 211, 212
Williford, W.O.: 221, 222
Wills, W.: 149
Wilson, D.B.: 244
Wilson, W.T.: 150
Wing, J.: 8, 9
Winman, F.: 77
Winnett, R.L.: 176
Witkin, M.J.: 11
Wolf, M.: 43
Wolff, W.: 77
Woods, D.: 43, 77
Woody, G.E.: 70
Wright, C.: 181, 228

Yates, B.T.: 248
Yeaton, W.H.: 69, 70, 131

Zakos, B.: 54
Zarcone, V.: 192, 207
Zasslow, M.: 231
Zillmer, E.W.: 41

Subject Index

Adaptation:
  client perceptions: 212–213
  community: 2–4, 199–214, 242
  in-program: 191
Adult status: 166, 215
Aggregate resident and staff characteristics: 2, 17, 116, 157–158, 167–172, 240–241
Aggressive behavior: 15, 65, 185–186, 243
Alcoholics Anonymous: 71, 91, 136, 208, 244–245, 250–251
Alcohol(ism) treatment programs: 71, 131–136, 207–208

Change:
  alcohol treatment program: 134
  clients' perception: 187
  health care system: 78, 244
  in community programs (COPES): 109, 112–113, 117–124
  in hospital programs (WAS): 60–67
  in programs: 4, 8, 37, 42, 45, 51, 53–58, 74, 85, 87–88, 138, 163, 235, 238–240
  life context: 250
  personality: 83–84
  process: 53–28, 125
  program climate: 174, 176
  social behavior: 73, 82–84, 185
  work environment: 230
  youth residential program: 125–130
Characteristics of Treatment Environments Scale: 23
Community adaptation and adjustment: 212–214
Community Oriented Programs Environment Scale (COPES): 17, 94–97, 234

adult residential program: 110–111
alcoholism treatment programs: 131–136
assessment/feedback process: 130
change: 109, 112–113, 117–124, 238
client empowerment: 210–211
community care home: 111–112
drug treatment programs: 137–139
Form E (Expectations): 187
Form I (Ideal): 105–108, 235
Form R (Real): 96
halfway house: 117–121
normative samples: 96–100
professional versus paraprofessional staff: 142–144
program descriptions: 113–116
program treatment model: 139–140
psychiatric and dual diagnosis programs: 140–142
psychometric criteria and characteristics: 95–96, 102–104
rehabilitation model: 122–124
staff reactions to feedback: 112–113
staff role and perceptions: 104–105
teaching family program: 121–122
United Kingdom sample: 100–102
youth residential program: 125–130
Community tenure rates: 200–206
Community versus hospital programs: 149–153
Congruence:
  actual-preferred environment: 87, 224–225
  client-group home manager: 209
  client-program: 216–225, 243
  patient-hospital staff: 87
  person-environment: 2
Coping:
  and treatment environments: 198, 242

behavior: 181–183
community adaptation: 199, 249
consonant styles: 178, 213
life context: 249–250
skills training: 225, 244
Cross-cultural comparisons: 33–34, 100

Disturbed patients:
children: 77, 227
community tenure: 201–203
group homes: 141, 151, 209–210
program expectation: 216–220
stepped model of care: 56
therapeutic communities: 55
treatment climates: 225
undifferentiated programs: 147
university hospital programs: 32–33
WAS profiles: 48, 81
Dropout:
and attrition rates: 188–194
correlation with patients' perceptions:
192–193, 201
Veterans' Resource Program: 123
Drug treatment programs: 104, 137–139

Estimated Omega Squared: 37, 103
Evaluating program descriptions: 113–
116
Expectations:
and patients' level of disturbance:
216–220, 234
clarity of: 50, 63, 66, 128, 132, 167,
175, 219
community: 250
in United Kingdom: 35
patients of program: 187
program/staff of patients: 83, 92, 106,
122, 167, 172, 198, 210, 213, 215,
224, 239, 241–243, 246
social interchange: 14–15, 216
unrealistic: 105
WAS: 24–26

Family Environment Scale (FES): 211
Feedback:
COPES: 94, 109, 112–113, 125, 128–
129, 130, 134
improving programs: 239–240
intentional social system: 83
staff-to-patient: 54
WAS: 45, 60–62, 65–66, 71, 72, 88

Group Environment Scale (GES): 77,
139
Group therapy: 12, 14, 57, 71, 82, 110,
114–115, 134, 168, 186, 220
Guidelines for writing program descriptions: 116

Halfway houses: 11, 53, 91–93, 96, 100,
114, 117–121, 131, 146, 177
Halo subscale:
COPES: 96
WAS: 26, 35–36
Health care workplace: 226–232
Helping behavior: 181, 183–184
Helping Scale: 183

Ideal treatment environment: 43, 70, 107,
124, 131, 209
Inmate Management Scale: 23
Insight-oriented programs: 79–81
Institutional context: 2, 17–18, 116, 157–
162, 172, 240–241
Intentional social systems model of care:
70, 82–88
Internal consistencies:
COPES: 96, 102, 106
WAS: 35–36, 43
Interpersonal behavior and adaption:
181–188
Intraclass correlations:
COPES: 114
WAS: 36, 38
Item-subscale correlations:
COPES: 96, 102, 106
WAS: 28, 35, 43

Job satisfaction: 56, 226

Milieu programs: 12, 15, 134–136, 236–
237
Moral treatment: 5–6, 10, 92, 124, 150,
233

Occupational therapy: 6, 84, 150, 151
Ownership: 17, 157, 159, 240

Perception of Ward Scales: 23
Personal development: 174–175, 204
Personal growth dimensions: 234–235,
239, 242
and age: 169

and community adjustment: 209, 211, 213
and community tenure rate: 203–204
and dropout rates: 192
and patients' level of disturbance: 216–217
and social climate: 159
and staff role: 104–105
in community programs: 101, 107, 117, 121, 136, 142–145
(COPES): 93, 96, 106–107
United Kingdom programs: 101, 107
in hospital programs: 39–40, 43, 49, 51, 53, 55, 61, 72, 78–79, 84–85, 87
(WAS): 28, 43, 60
United Kingdom programs: 34, 43
Physical design/features: 2, 16–18, 59, 100, 113, 116, 157–158, 162–165, 172, 174–175, 221–222, 227, 240–241
Policies and services: 2, 100, 116, 157–158, 165–167, 172, 240–241
Policy and Program Information Form: 165
Profile stability:
COPES: 103
WAS: 36–37, 43

Quality of life: 179, 211, 252

Relationship dimensions: 235, 237
and age: 39
and community adjustment: 209, 211
and community tenure rate: 203–204
and dropout rates: 192, 198
and patients' level of disturbance: 216–217
and social climate: 159
and staff role: 105
in community programs: 99, 102, 110–111, 117, 121, 123, 135–136, 141–142
(COPES): 93, 96, 106–107
United Kingdom programs: 101, 107–108
in hospital programs: 33, 49, 51, 55, 61, 72, 76–79, 84, 180
(WAS): 28, 36, 43
United Kingdom programs: 43

Satisfaction: 3, 56, 72, 130, 163, 177–181, 184, 188, 211, 221, 226
Self-confidence: 179–181
Size: 17, 33–34, 51, 81, 99, 100, 116, 119, 157, 160–161, 175, 189, 240
Social Climate Scales: 40
Social integration and community living skills: 209–212
Social interaction: 9, 14, 158, 164, 170, 174, 185, 209, 212, 215–216
Staffing: 17, 33–34, 46, 51, 81, 116, 135–136, 157, 162, 189, 240
Staff morale: 7–8, 54, 56, 65, 85, 100, 163, 165, 226, 228, 231, 239
Staff role: 12, 41, 82, 104–105
Symptom reduction and psychosocial functioning: 207–209
System maintenance dimensions (staff control): 150–152, 234–235, 238, 242
and age: 39, 169
and community adjustment: 211
and community tenure rate: 203–204, 206
and dropout rates: 192–193, 198
and institutional context: 160–162
and patients' level of disturbance: 216–217, 220
and social climate: 159, 166, 168, 171–172
and staff role: 104–105
in community programs: 100, 111, 117, 120–121, 123, 136, 139–145, 147, 151
(COPES): 93, 96, 107
United Kingdom programs: 101–102
in hospital programs: 33, 40, 49, 51, 55, 61, 66, 72, 76, 78–79, 84–85, 87, 181
(WAS): 28, 30, 36, 43, 60
United Kingdom programs: 34, 43
staff control: 13, 16, 30, 38, 41, 43, 47, 54, 57, 59, 64, 74, 122, 126, 128, 132, 139–140, 178–179, 182, 184–186, 208, 213, 227–228

Task groups: 12–13, 82, 87, 250
Therapeutic community programs:
and change: 64, 122–123, 239
children's programs: 77–78

client perceptions: 194
community tenure: 205
design: 55
dropout rate: 192
forensic hospitals: 45
implementation: 74–76, 237
milieu-oriented: 15
problems: 65–66
psychiatric & dual diagnosis
    programs: 141
short-stay programs: 75
social rehabilitation: 11–12
substance abuse: 72–73, 137
symptom reduction & psychosocial
    functioning: 207
typology: 78, 145–146, 235
Therapists: 8, 9, 63
Total institutions: 8
Treatment goals: 7, 12, 47, 70, 111, 120,
    204–206, 236, 238, 240, 245
Treatment outcomes: 15, 18, 23, 65, 70,
    130, 177, 188, 192, 193, 208, 212–
    213, 220, 238, 243–245, 249–251
Turnover rates: 194–196
Typology of programs:
    community programs: 145–148
    hospital programs: 78–81

Ward Atmosphere Scale (WAS): 16, 25–
    30, 234
acute admission and rehabilitation

programs: 70–72
as a teaching aid: 60–61
assessment/feedback process: 86–88,
    130
change: 53–59, 61–64, 66–67, 235,
    238
children's programs: 77–78
community tenure: 201
demographic characteristics: 39–40
dropout rate: 189–190
Form I (Ideal): 42–44, 64, 235
Form R (Real): 25–30
inpatient and day hospital programs:
    64–66
medical programs: 76–77
patient satisfaction: 179–180
personality and role factors: 40–43
program descriptions: 45–53
psychometric criteria and characteris-
    tics: 27–28, 35–38
staff education: 57
state hospital programs: 31–32, 48–50
substance abuse programs: 72–74
therapeutic community programs: 55,
    74–75
United Kingdom programs: 33–35,
    43–44
university hospital programs: 32–33,
    45–48
VA hospital programs: 31–32, 50–51
Work stress: 231